The Nautilus Nutrition Book

Ellington Darden, Ph.D.

Photography by Scott LeGear

Contemporary Books, Inc.
Chicago

Library of Congress Cataloging in Publication Data

Darden, Ellington, 1943-
   The Nautilus nutrition book.

   Bibliography: p.
   Includes index.
   1. Nutrition.   I. Title.
TX353.D23   641.1   81-65186
ISBN 0-8092-5891-9   AACR2
ISBN 0-8092-5890-0 (pbk.)

Published by Contemporary Books, Inc.
180 North Michigan Avenue, Chicago, Illinois 60601
Manufactured in the United States of America
Library of Congress Catalog Card Number: 81-65186
International Standard Book Number: 0-8092-5891-9 (cloth)
                                                    0-8092-5890-0 (paper)

Published simultaneously in Canada by
Beaverbooks, Ltd.
150 Lesmill Road
Don Mills, Ontario M3B 2T5
Canada

contents

foreword

If you want accurate information about nutrition, select your sources carefully. Misinformation does not carry a warning label!

Most newspapers and magazines will publish sensational claims about nutrition without attempting to judge their accuracy. "Health food" magazines deliberately slant their articles to promote the products of their advertisers. And most nutrition books intended for the general public are written by leading quacks.

Most "nutrition experts" who appear on radio or television talk shows have no scientific training at all. They are store owners or other health food industry representatives who want to sell you something. Instead of telling you that a balanced diet can easily supply all the nutrients you need, they say that everyone needs supplements. Instead of telling you that the American food supply is the safest in the world, they claim that it contains "too many chemicals." Instead of promoting moderation as a basic principle of nutrition, they suggest that "if some is good, more is better."

Few people realize how skillfully promoters of quackery are doing their jobs. People who answer ads for phony reducing gadgets or dietary schemes think that the ads must be true or somehow "they wouldn't be allowed." Mothers who give their children vitamin pills rarely stop to think about whether they are needed. Nor do athletes taking huge amounts of protein or other food supplements think of themselves as susceptible to quackery. They are just imitating the habits of their favorite champions.

As far as we know, no magazine has ever published an in-depth analysis of sports fads and fakes. A few years ago, a female weight lifter—"The World's Strongest Woman"—told *Sports Illustrated* magazine that, at the peak of her training, she took close to 200 vitamin pills a day. Concerned that her story would encourage budding athletes to waste money or endanger their health, I sent letters to each of the sixty-one publishers, editors, and writers listed on the magazine's masthead, suggesting that the scientific facts of the matter be explored. When nothing came of this effort, my committee and several prominent medical writers contacted *Sport, Family Health,* and a large number of popular magazines. Not one was interested.

Why not?

In some cases, the answer is money. Sensation increases readership, and vitamin companies advertise—a lot. In other cases, it is fear of controversy. Readers who regard nutrition as a form of religion tend to get nasty when their myths are criticized—so why look for trouble?

The imbalance in the media could improve if the scientific community made a concerted effort to speak out against quackery, but most scientists are uneasy about entering public controversy.

Not so Ellington Darden. Highly trained in nutrition, physical education, and communication, he is one of the dozen or so individuals in America who are willing to confront quackery wherever they encounter it.

The Nautilus Nutrition Book is designed not only to provide basic facts, but also to expose misinformation—for athletes and nonathletes alike. Use it in good health!

Stephen Barrett, M.D.
Chairman, Board of Directors
Lehigh Valley Committee
Against Health Fraud, Inc.

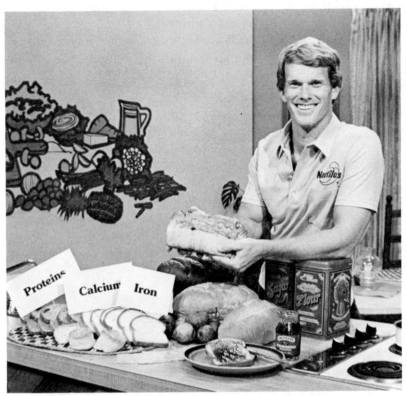

Ellington Darden, Ph.D.

preface

The Nautilus Nutrition Book does not promote food fads. But it does tell how to stay well-nourished through sensible eating.

It does not present a new diet for fast weight loss. But it does present scientifically based steps for removing body fat and keeping it off permanently.

The book does not say that Americans are being poisoned to death by eating food additives and pesticides. It does not berate the food industry, the Department of Agriculture, or the Food and Drug Administration. Instead, it emphasizes that we do have excellent, safe food in this country.

This is not the popular position to take. It is much easier to take the poisons-in-the-food stance, to offer natural organic alternatives, and to stress the need for supplements.

Several factors put me in a unique position to write The Nautilus Nutrition Book.

As Director of Research for Nautilus Sports/Medical Industries, I have been involved in the development of Nautilus almost from the ground floor. I have spent hundreds of hours with the man who developed Nautilus machines. Observing, listening, questioning, and discussing the human body with Arthur Jones has been most meaningful to me.

I first met him at the 1970 National Powerlifting Contest in New Orleans. He exhibited his pullover machine and talked with interested people concerning Nautilus training. Later that year I visited the Nautilus Fitness Center in DeLand, Florida. There Arthur Jones put me through my initial Nautilus workout. I was impressed with Jones and with his machines.

Two years later, after finishing a postdoctoral study in the Food and Nutrition Department at Florida State University, I went to work for Nautilus Sports/Medical Industries. Since that time I have been amazed at its rapid growth and development from a single Nautilus Fitness Center in 1970 to more than 2,400 in 1981. An estimated 3.5 million people now regularly exercise on Nautilus equipment.

Nautilus has revolutionized the fitness industry. The revolution occurred for several reasons. One, the general public was tired of false claims about quick and easy ways to get into shape. Two, Nautilus was not afraid to tell people the truth. Three, Nautilus works. It works because it is based on the physics and chemistry of the human body.

In the summer of 1980, *The Nautilus Book: An Illustrated Guide to Physical Fitness the Nautilus Way* was published. Because of its wide acceptance, more people than ever were introduced to the benefits of training on Nautilus equipment. But more important, these people began to learn about the research and logic behind the Nautilus machines.

The time is ripe for a similar revolution to take place in nutrition. The public is not being helped by lies about crash diets that do not work, magic foods for every ill, and the dangers of eating processed foods. It is time for someone to stand up and tell the truth.

That is why *The Nautilus Nutrition Book* was written. Nutrition, like exercise, can be reduced to physics and to chemistry of the human body. Nothing is more logical than physics and chemistry. These sciences indicate that exercise and nutrition must be balanced with the requirements of the human body. Nautilus exercise is balanced exercise. Nautilus nutrition is balanced nutrition. Balanced exercise and balanced nutrition make a perfect marriage.

Of equal importance to this book is the time I spent with Dr. Harold E. Schendel. For three years Dr. Schendel was my major professor in the Food and Nutrition Department at Florida State University.

When I entered graduate school at Florida State in 1968, I was a confirmed food faddist. I consumed massive amounts of protein supplements each day. I took vitamin B_{12} for endurance, wheat germ oil for energy, garlic for purifying the blood, kelp tablets for muscle definition, and vitamin B_6 for strength. At the same time, I avoided white bread, carbonated drinks, ice cream, and most other carbohydrate-rich foods. I was convinced that this dietary program would help me become a superior athlete.

Where did I get these beliefs? The majority came from physical fitness and health magazines. According to these publications, most recent champions had followed such a program. I never questioned these concepts until I entered graduate school. In fact, I kept trying to find new ways or more concentrated protein supplements to be certain that I was consuming more than 300 grams of protein per day.

After I met Dr. Schendel, we spent many hours discussing how various foods and eating habits might affect athletic performance and health in general. Dr. Schendel disagreed with most of my nutritional concepts and did not believe that my special eating habits were necessary, beneficial, or even safe. According to him, an athlete did *not* require large amounts of vitamins, proteins, or any special foods.

Dr. Schendel did not convince me. After all, his knowledge was mostly theoretical, but I was actually eating a special diet and "knew" about its value. I was following the methods of champions and was not about to change my athletic training program because of any university professor or research done on rats. Rather than argue, however, Dr. Schendel suggested that I experiment on myself to determine whether an athlete in hard training could actually use the massive amounts of protein I was eating.

For two months, I kept precise records of my dietary intake, of my energy expenditure, and of my general well-being. My protein intake was varied from less than 100 grams per day to more than 380 grams, most of this obtained from a 90% protein powder. All my urine was collected and analyzed to see whether the protein I ate was being used by my body or merely broken down and excreted through my kidneys.

The result of this study startled me. According to the Recommended Dietary Allowances, my protein need for a body weight of 215 pounds was 77 grams per day. To my surprise, whenever I consumed more than this amount, the excess was excreted. My weight remained relatively constant and I noted no difference in strength regardless of the amount of protein consumed. In fact, when I went off my massive protein diet (relieving my body of the burden of metabolizing the excess protein), I experienced a surge of energy.

Furthermore, when I consumed more than the Recommended Dietary Allowances of various vitamins and minerals, excess amounts of these substances were also excreted rather than used by my body. It took a personal experience to undo the brainwashing I had undergone during my early years as an athlete.

"A single experience," says Arthur Jones, "can trigger a thought pattern that leads out of a blind alley . . . and having emerged into the light, you then have the opportunity to examine the involved factors."

This statement certainly describes my initial meetings with both Arthur Jones and Harold Schendel. In the ensuing years, I have studied carefully the many factors that make up proper exercise and nutrition.

Today, I understand why nutrition for optimum performance requires no more than a well-balanced diet composed of foods that are readily available at grocery stores and supermarkets. The only people who benefit from expensive food supplements are those who sell them.

As I travel the country conducting Nautilus lectures and workshops, I notice that people are concerned about nutrition. They have hundreds of questions. They want to know about vitamin C and vitamin E. Which foods produce quick energy? Is additional protein necessary for building strength? How many calories are used during a Nautilus workout? Are natural foods better than processed foods? Which foods should be avoided on a reducing diet? They ask questions about sugar, salt, and fast foods; questions about losing and gaining weight. Questions, questions, and more questions.

Sometimes when I lecture I am not sure I am reaching the audience. But when the questions come thick and furiously at the conclusion of my presentation, I know I am stimulating the listeners to *think*.

I like questions. *The Nautilus Nutrition Book*, therefore, is a book of questions and answers.

Ellington Darden, Ph.D.
Lake Helen, FL
September 17, 1981

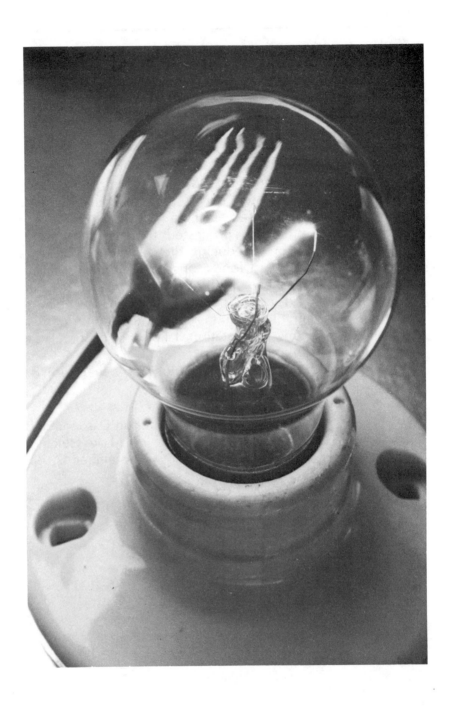

I.

NUTRITION IN ACTION

1

determining nutritional status

NUTRITION DEFINED

Q. *Much has been written about nutrition. Exactly what is it?*

A. Nutrition is a science. Like all sciences, it is a body of systematized facts that have been established according to scientific methods.

Nutrition belongs to the group of natural sciences or those that concern nature and the physical world. Natural sciences may be divided into pure and applied sciences. Pure sciences include mathematics, physics, chemistry, and biology. Those described as applied are engineering, medicine, nutrition, agriculture, and geology.

To some people, nutrition refers to the preparation and service of tasty foods in an attractive manner. Although nutrition begins with food, it surely does not end there. To others, nutrition refers more to various agricultural practices used in the growth and development of healthy, marketable live-

2

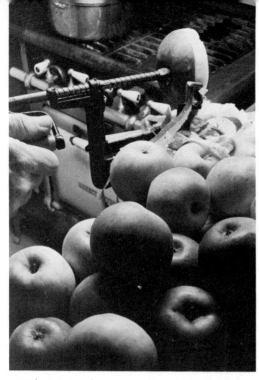

Nutrition, in part, deals with the preparation of wholesome food at home. Applesauce made in the old-fashioned way usually involved washing, coring, peeling, slicing, cooking, spicing, cooling, and storage. Many people still enjoy the lengthy process of preparing foods at home from scratch.

stock. To other people, it refers to cell processes and how cells receive their required nutrients. Actually, it includes all of these.

Nutrition is both a scientific discipline and a biological process. For the purpose of this book, the word *nutrition* is defined as *the study of food and how the body uses it*. Nutrition is a process by which food is ingested and digested and its nutrients are absorbed and distributed to cells in all parts of the body. Here they are either used and extra amounts stored, or they are excreted along with the unabsorbed food debris and the waste products of the body processes. The attainment of nutritional status is dependent on the performance of many integrated systems in the body.

This nutritional process may be successful, or it may be faulty in varying degrees at different points of the digestion and excretion process. Faulty nutrition or malnutrition may result from eating too little or too much food, from consuming the wrong kinds of food, or from a functional failure in one or more systems of the body.

Various terms have been used by laymen to describe the quality of an individual's nutritional state. Three general categories, however, are used by nutritionists to describe the nutritional status of a subject: undernutrition, optimum nutrition, and overnutrition. The first and last of these states also can be described as types of malnutrition. Obviously, undernutrition of one or all nutrients may also lead to ill health and disease. Today, far more Americans suffer from ill health due to overnutrition than from deficiency states or undernutrition. More Americans die from heart disease, a problem of overnutrition, than from all other diseases combined.

Although food is the basic factor in preventing malnutrition, an individual must learn how to select the right foods, to prepare them correctly, and to consume them in the proper amount and at the right time in order to achieve optimum nutrition.

NUTRITIONAL STATUS

Q. *How can an individual measure his own nutritional status?*

Nutrition also involves the advances in food technology that allow the modern cook the convenience of purchasing foods that have been prepared under controlled conditions. For example, at a large citrus processing plant, oranges are washed, cut, juiced, tested, blended, and retested for flavor. The juice is then dispensed into plastic containers that are immediately sealed, frozen, and stored where it awaits shipment. The entire process is performed efficiently by stainless steel machines under standardized conditions that guarantee minimum nutrient losses. Furthermore, modern technology has found a use for the remaining citrus rind and pulp. The leftovers are pulverized and used for cattle feed.

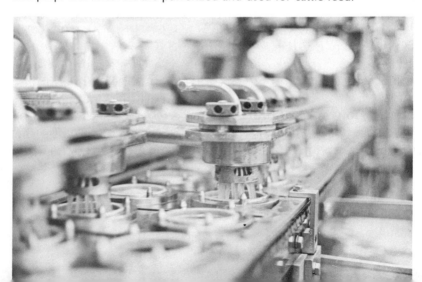

A. A general estimate of nutritional status can be made by the individual after analyzing his own eating habits. Details on how to do this are presented later in the chapter. If a person feels well and eats well, however, it can be assumed that his nutritional status is satisfactory.

To make a thorough assessment of a person's nutritional status it is necessary to view the task as a series of evaluations applied to the body as a whole or to body areas sensitive to nutritional measurements. Such evaluations require sophisticated techniques. These techniques are designed for use by specialists in various scientific fields.

Q. *What are some of the techniques that are used to measure nutritional status?*

A. Perhaps the first step in the assessment of a person's nutritional status is a general physical examination and dietary evaluation. Physicians are aware that many nutritional deficiencies may be expressed by some of the following superficial signs and symptoms: stiff and brittle hair; abnormally dry and rough skin; dry, dull, lusterless eyes with irritated lids; a deep red and fissured tongue; spongy and bleeding gums; and lips that are swollen, chapped, and cracked at the corners.

The second step in the assessment of nutritional status should be the measurement of the body's ability to perform its various functions; for example, color vision, vision in dim light, heart function, and work capacity.

Since these gross clinical signs and functions are easy to observe, they are often used in making the initial estimate of an individual's nutritional status. They are also general signs of ill health and do not necessarily indicate malnutrition. Malnutrition can also be provoked by nondietary factors such as infection or by faulty digestion, absorption, utilization, or elimination.

The diagram on page 6 by the well-known British nutritionist, Dr. H. M. Sinclair, points out that a person's physical well-being is composed of many interrelated factors:

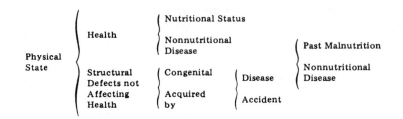

This diagram indicates the complex nature of body condition and the difficulty in assessing it.

BLOOD AND URINE TESTS

Q. *Would blood and urine tests be helpful?*

A. Yes, blood and urine tests offer a more precise but expensive way of assessing nutritional status. Such measurements reveal the status of nutrients circulating in the blood or being excreted in the urine. These data can be judged to be normal by comparison with measurements from healthy, well-nourished individuals of the same sex, age, physical development, and activity.

HAIR ANALYSIS

Q. *Can hair analysis reveal a person's nutritional state?*

A. Many medical authorities warn fitness-minded people to *beware* of hair analysis. For example, Dr. Charles Butterworth, Chairman of the Department of Nutritional Science at the University of Alabama Medical Center, says: "Hair analysis sounds like a good idea, but it isn't. Despite the appeal of simplicity, there are too many errors: Things you eat today can show up much later, a hair from one part of the head won't be the same as one from another area, and there is no established method. Different people can use different methods to produce different results."

Hair analysis may have some use in the diagnosis of poison-

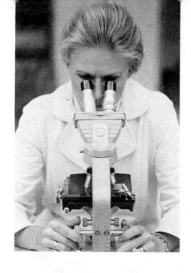

Laboratory tests can use small samples of blood and urine for evaluation of nutritional status.

ing by heavy metals such as lead and mercury. But it is of limited value in determining a person's nutritional status. Fitness-minded individuals should be skeptical of professional people who use hair analysis as the basis for prescribing food supplements.

BODY-FAT EVALUATION

Q. *Does nutritional status include desirable height-weight and body-fat analysis?*

A. Height, weight, and body fat are factors to consider in determining a person's nutritional status.

The problem with the traditional height-weight charts is that they do not distinguish between the weight of excess fat, which is unhealthy, and the weight of large muscles, which may be desirable for athletes. The charts are simply averages of the general population. A better method of determining the fatness of an individual would be to obtain a measurement of body fat.

Several methods have been used to measure body fat, namely X rays, specific gravity, potassium 40, and skin-fold thickness. Skin-fold thickness is the easiest and most popular method of assessing body fat. The thickness of a fold of skin in various areas of the body is measured with skin-fold calipers. Such data can then be translated into percentage of body fat. Although these data are not perfect or totally precise, they do give a better indication of amount of body fat

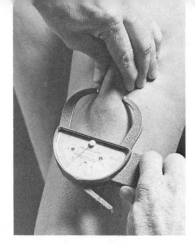

Skinfold calipers, properly used by experts, provide a better indication of an individual's body fatness or leanness than height–weight charts.

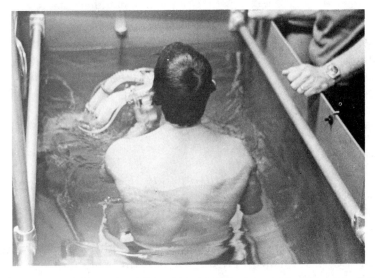

Underwater weighings (specific gravity) of the human body, compared to skinfold measurements, offer a more precise method of estimating fatness and leanness. But such weighings are also more complex, expensive, and time consuming. (Photo by Ellington Darden)

than mere body weight and height. Typically, the amount of body fat varies with age and sex. In general, it is greatest in infancy and diminishes in childhood and increases again during adolescence. Research indicates that girls and women normally have more body fat than do boys and men. An abnormally great or small amount of body fat is related to poor nutritional status.

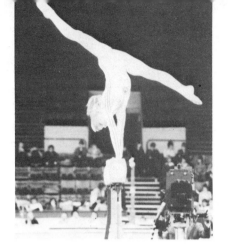

Women who participate skillfully in gymnastics usually have a very low percentage of body fat. (Photo by David Ponsonby)

More than 20% of the body weight of most Americans is fat. And, as expected, athletes have a smaller percentage of fat than nonathletes. The table on page 10 shows the results of a study recently completed on Czechoslovakian athletes. Most of these athletes have a small amount of body fat. In fact, seldom does a successful male athlete have more than 12% body fat.

BASIC FOUR FOOD GROUPS

Q. *Is there a magic formula for healthful eating?*
A. The closest thing to a magic formula is this advice: eat a variety of foods and do not eat too much of anything.

In the 1940s the U.S. Department of Agriculture devised what they called the Basic Seven to explain the variety of foods needed in the diet. They listed milk, meats, citrus fruits, green and yellow vegetables, other fruits and vegetables, bread and cereals, butter and margarine. Actually, this list was a condensed version of the Basic Eleven, which ruled the nutritional world earlier in the century.

In an effort to simplify the nutritional guidelines even further, the Department of Agriculture introduced the Basic Four in 1958. Making wise selections from these four basic food groups is an individual's best bet for variety and balance.

Body Weight and Fatness of 10 Men and
10 Women Champions in Different Sports*

MEN	Weight (lbs.)	% Body Fat
1. Gymnastics	148.7	4.5
2. Marathon runners	135.7	6.1
3. Weight lifting	170.3	6.2
4. Racing cycling	155.8	6.2
5. Tennis	138.2	7.3
6. Volleyball	174.7	7.5
7. Table tennis	128.7	9.2
8. Basketball	215.8	11.7
9. Ice hockey	148.1	14.8
10. Greco-Roman wrestling	227.0	19.0
WOMEN		
1. Gymnastics	122.3	8.3
2. Gymnastics	117.7	10.2
3. High jump	136.8	10.3
4. 10 m diving	110.0	12.4
5. Skiing 10 km	120.1	13.5
6. Swimming	153.6	13.8
7. Ice skating	128.3	15.3
8. Tennis	137.5	18.2
9. Table tennis	115.3	18.3
10. Shot put and discus	179.7	19.7

* From *Nutrition and Athletic Performance* by Ellington Darden, Pasadena, California: The Athletic Press, 1976, p. 29.

Milk Group

Nearly everyone should have some milk or milk product every day for protein, calcium, phosphorus, and certain vitamins. This group includes whole and skimmed milk, buttermilk, yogurt, cottage cheese, ice cream, and cheese. At least two servings from the milk group are needed each day.

Meat Group

Included in the meat group are beef, veal, pork, liver, heart, kidney, fish, poultry, eggs, dried beans, nuts, and lentils. Two servings daily are desirable to ensure that an individual gets adequate amounts of protein, iron, and some of the vitamins. Vegetarians can readily get protein of good nutritional quality and quantity by consuming extra milk, cheese, and eggs.

Bread and Cereal Group

Enriched or whole-grain breads and cereals provide energy-giving carbohydrates, many vitamins and minerals, and a source of protein. Four or more servings should be included each day.

Fruit and Vegetable Group

Selections from this group should amount to four servings a day, with both green and yellow fruits and vegetables included. Fruits and vegetables are excellent sources of carbohydrates, vitamins, minerals, fiber, and water.

Other Foods

The Basic Four foods have serious functions to perform: the jobs of building, maintenance, and repair. But what of other foods, such as candy, soft drinks, butter, margarine, salad dressings, and snacks? Should they be written off or sacrificed? As long as the basic nutritional needs are met, everyone should have access to this group—at least a limited access.

All foods in this group are primarily sources of energy. By themselves they cannot sustain life, but they can add flavor and variety to meals and add to the joy of living. When large amounts of fat must be lost, this group is the best place for an individual to make cuts.

MEAL RECORDS

Q. *How does a fitness-minded individual know if he is eating correctly?*

A. Until a person keeps a daily record of his eating habits, he probably does not realize how much of particular foods he consumes. In this respect, an individual is urged to record the details of his diet. He will need to record how much of each food he consumes for several days, both on weekdays and on weekends. This will make a person aware of the frequency of eating, the quality and quantity of the food consumed, and eating habits that need improvement.

Guidelines for how to evaluate present dietary habits are presented on the following pages.

1. Select a day that is representative of typical eating habits (usually a weekday).

2. Write down what is eaten at each meal and between meals.

3. Record food quantities in food groups columns. For example, if a person ate the following breakfast:

   ½ cup orange juice
   1 egg
   2 slices buttered toast
   1 cup milk

he would record as follows:

	Milk Group	Meat Group	Fruits and Vegetables	Bread and Cereal	Additional Foods
Breakfast	1	1	1	2	2

Record the other foods consumed throughout the day in a similar manner on the Typical One-Day Meal Record table. Transfer these total amounts to the Food Scoreboard that applies most closely to the daily energy requirements.

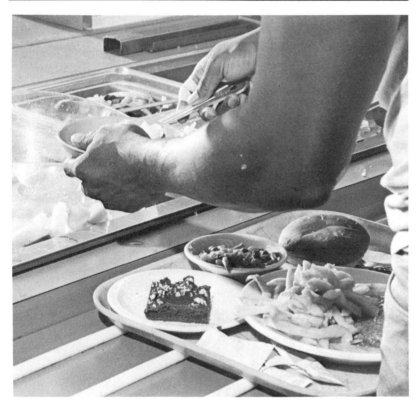

The basis of good nutrition is eating a variety of foods from the Basic Four Food Groups. No single food group supplies all the essential nutrients in proper proportions to maintain health.

Typical One-Day Meal Record

Food Groups

Meal	Milk Group (cups)	Meat Group (servings)	Fruits and Vegetables (servings)	Bread and Cereal (servings)	Additional Foods (fats, candy, desserts, soft drinks, snacks)
Breakfast					
Midmorning Snack					
Lunch					
Afternoon Snack					
Dinner					
Evening Snack					
Totals					

Food Scoreboard (Approximately 2,500 calories)

Recommended Food	Goal	Score
Milk	3 cups	_____
Meat	5 ounces	_____
Fruits and Vegetables	8 servings	_____
Fruits	6 servings	_____
Vegetables	2 servings	_____
Bread	8 servings	_____
	4 with jelly	_____
Other	2 desserts	_____
	2 teaspoons oil	_____

Foods to Add	Foods to Cut Down On
_____	_____
_____	_____
_____	_____

Food Scoreboard (Approximately 3,750 calories)

Recommended Food	Goal	Score
Milk	4½ cups	_____
Meat	7½ ounces	_____
Fruits and Vegetables	12 servings	_____
Fruits	9 servings	_____
Vegetables	3 servings	_____
Bread	12 servings	_____
	6 with jelly	_____
Other	3 desserts	_____
	3 teaspoons oil	_____

Foods to Add	Foods to Cut Down On
_____	_____
_____	_____
_____	_____

Food Scoreboard (Approximately 5,000 calories)

Recommended Foods	Goal	Scoreboard
Milk	6 cups	_____
Meat	10 ounces	_____
Fruits and Vegetables	16 servings	_____
Fruits	12 servings	_____
Vegetables	4 servings	_____
Bread	16 servings	_____
	8 with jelly	_____
Other	4 desserts	_____
	4 teaspoons oil	_____

Foods to Add	Foods to Cut Down On
_____	_____
_____	_____
_____	_____

Individuals who wish to determine more precisely the composition of their diet may do so after acquiring these two books:

1. *Composition of Foods: Raw, Processed, Prepared,* Agriculture Handbook No. 8, supplied by the Agriculture Research Service, U.S. Department of Agriculture, Washington, DC.

2. *Nutritive Value of Foods,* Home and Garden Bulletin No. 72, U.S. Department of Agriculture, Washington, DC.

These books are inexpensive and may be obtained from the extension service of the state university or from the Superintendent of Documents, U.S. Government Printing Office, Washington, DC 20402.

MEAL-PLANNING GUIDELINES

Q. *What is the basis for the food scoreboard guidelines?*

A. The food scoreboards were developed according to the basic diet described by the Food and Nutrition Board of the National Research Council. This diet consists of two to four cups of milk a day, two servings of meat, four or more servings of fruits and vegetables, and four or more servings from the bread group. By following this procedure, a fitness-minded individual will be able to test the nutritional quality or adequacy of his diet.

Recent research shows that the average American consumes more than 3,400 calories a day. Of these calories, 45% come from carbohydrates, 12% from proteins, and 43% from fats. Nutrition and medical authorities agree that Americans consume too many calories. These calories are provided primarily by refined sugars and fat.

Americans consume many pastries and other desserts, foods fried in fat, and much beef. The average American eats more than 100 grams of protein each day, primarily in the form of meat and dairy products. Although these foods contain high quality protein, amounts eaten in excess of body needs are converted to fat.

Authorities also recommend that the fat content of the American diet should be reduced to approximately 30–35%. The optimum diet for health should look like the following as far as proportions are concerned:

	Fat	Protein	Carbohydrate
Average American Diet	43%	12%	45%
Optimum Diet for Health	30—35%	12—15%	55—58%

Using these guidelines, diets for three energy levels have been developed: diets that provide 2,500, 3,750, and 5,000 calories per day. The diets are described by listing the appropriate amounts of the food groups, as well as their nutrient content.

Total Servings of Foods in Daily Meal Schedules

Approximate Calories	Whole Milk	Meat or Equivalent	Fruit	Veg.	Bread	Other
2,500	3 cups	5 ounces	6 ser.	2 ser.	8 ser. 4 with jelly	2 desserts 2 tsp. oil
3,750	4½ cups	7½ ounces	9 ser.	3 ser.	12 ser. 6 with jelly	3 desserts 3 tsp. oil
5,000	6 cups	10 ounces	12 ser.	4 ser.	16 ser. 8 with jelly	4 desserts 4 tsp. oil

Approximate Nutrient Content of Daily Meal Schedules

Approximate Calories	Fat		Protein		Carbohydrate	
	Grams	% Total Calories	Grams	% Total Calories	Grams	% Total Calories
2,500	70	28	79	13	374	59
3,750	105	28	118	13	561	59
5,000	140	28	158	13	748	59

The nutrient content of these daily schedules is almost the same as the Optimum Diet for Health. An extra percentage point has been added for the athlete in protein and carbohydrate foods and two have been deducted from the fat sources. This will benefit the athlete's performance.

The daily meal schedules were developed for three energy levels: 2,500, 3,750, and 5,000 calories. From these three diets, a fitness-minded individual should be able to plan his own special diet. For example, both the 135-pound golfer and the 110-pound female gymnast might require 2,500 calories a day. On the other hand, the 225-pound football player should probably consume close to 5,000 calories as should the 165-pound swimmer in rigorous training. In between these athletes is the 175-pound weight lifter/bodybuilder who would require around 3,750 calories per day.

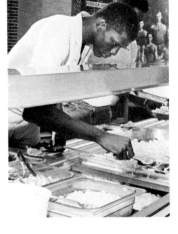

The ideal diet for an athlete should consist of 58% carbohydrates, 28% fats, and 13% proteins. The athlete needs additional energy, which can be obtained most efficiently from carbohydrate-rich foods such as fruits, vegetables, and bread.

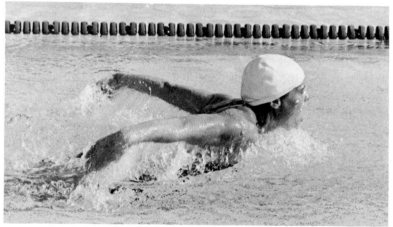

Swimming is a demanding sport. Many competitive swimmers must consume more than 5,000 calories per day during rigorous training.

RECOMMENDED ALLOWANCES

Q. *What does RDA mean?*

A. RDA stands for Recommended Dietary Allowance. These allowances (see Appendix A) are set by the Food and Nutrition Board of the National Research Council, National Academy of Sciences. Beginning in 1943, the National Research Council defined recommended allowances for the various dietary essentials for people of different ages. These standards, the Recommended Dietary Allowances (RDAs), represent not only the most authoritative estimates of recommended dietary intakes in the United States, but also the most up-to-date body of expert opinion available. The RDAs do not remain fixed over time. They are revised periodically in keeping with the best current scientific information about human nutritional needs.

Q. *Are the RDAs a good standard for determining the amount of nutrients required by athletes or individuals training on Nautilus equipment?*
A. The RDAs are listed according to the age and sex of healthy subjects living in the United States. These recommendations provide for the maintenance of excellent nutritional status and therefore are recommended as goals for the nutrient intake of all healthy Americans. Although the RDAs are based on minimum daily requirements, they also include a very ample margin of safety.

In the words of the Food and Nutrition Board, the RDAs "are meant to afford a margin of sufficiency above minimal requirements and are planned to provide a buffer against the needs of various stresses and to make possible other potential improvements of growth and function." Hence, the RDAs were designed to provide for maintenance of good nutrition not only for the average person but for *all* healthy persons, including athletes. It is conceivable that the stresses imposed by a vigorous conditioning program may exceed those provided by the RDAs, but such a situation would be very rare and only temporary. This explains why it is not justifiable for an athlete to consume a diet that is double or triple the RDAs by using multivitamin, protein, or mineral supplements.

An individual must use judgment in using the RDAs to evaluate the adequacy of his dietary intake. Failure to meet them should not be equated with malnutrition. It should be remembered that the RDAs are not requirements but generous allowances. When a person falls one-third below the RDA of a particular nutrient over a period of several weeks or more, he should find out why and make the necessary corrections in his eating habits.

The ultimate evaluation of an individual's nutritional status requires more than casual observation. Feeling below par is not sufficient evidence to justify the conclusion that a person is malnourished. Inadequate rest, illness, or emotional stresses can also rob people of their vitality. If a fitness-minded individual achieves the nutrient levels recommended by the Food and Nutrition Board, however, he can be assured of being well-nourished unless he has some physical abnormality or disease.

Q. *What is meant when the label of a food product says that one serving of the food supplies a certain proportion of the U.S. RDA of a particular nutrient?*

A. U.S. RDAs are the Food and Drug Administration's simplified version of the Recommended *Daily Allowances* set by the Food and Nutrition Board in 1968. The Recommended *Dietary* Allowances are abbreviated simply *RDAs* and should not be confused with the U.S. RDAs.

If a food is fortified with a nutrient or if a specific claim is made for a food, then nutritional labeling is required. Nutritional labeling must include information specifying, per serving size, the amount of protein, carbohydrate, and fat in grams; the number of calories; and the percent of the U.S. RDA fulfilled by seven vitamins and minerals. Information for 12 other vitamins and minerals and for cholesterol, fatty acids, and sodium content is optional.

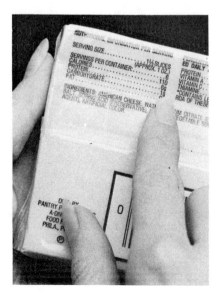

Today's consumer can judge the quality of many foods by comparing the nutrient composition on the labels.

BALANCED NUTRITION

Q. *The word* balance *is used in many ways in nutrition, such as in* balanced diet, caloric balance, vitamin and mineral balance. *What does it mean?*

A. The term *balanced diet* is a phrase that refers to a diet providing all the nutrients required by a person depending on his sex, age, activity, and physiological condition. Since no single food provides all of the fifty or more required nutrients in the proper amount, the balanced diet is usually made up of many different foods. It is often said to be a mixed diet.

The most noteworthy efforts to simplify the achievement of a balanced diet have been the development of the Recommended Dietary Allowances and the grouping of foods. Selection of foods from each of the Basic Four in the recommended amounts will provide a balanced or adequate diet.

When the term *balance* is used in phrases like *caloric balance* and *calcium balance*, it refers to intake versus output. Again the goal is to supply the body's requirements by replac-

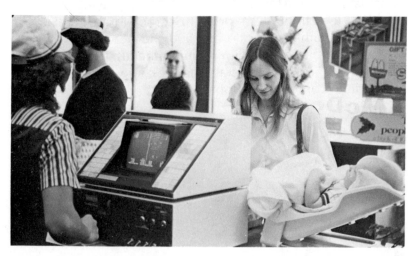

The goal of balanced nutrition is to supply all the nutrients required by a person without adding excessive body fat. Much is dependent, however, on the age and sex of the individual. A child, for example, requires different nutrient balance than an adult. And a young mother needs a degree of balance that is different from an older woman.

ing the nutrients used up or lost from the body without storing any great "excess baggage." A person is in caloric balance when the number of calories consumed equals the number expended. On the other hand, an individual would be in positive caloric balance when he is gaining weight due to storage of fat.

At some times it is desirable to be in a positive balance for certain nutrients, while at other times it is best to be in a negative balance. At still other times it is best to be in equilibrium. For example, a person should be in a negative caloric balance in order to lose fat, in a positive calcium balance during bone growth or healing, and in equilibrium for most nutrients in adulthood.

MEAL SIZE

Q. *What proportion of the daily caloric need should be consumed with each meal?*

A. The usual meal pattern for most people in the United States is a light breakfast and a moderate lunch followed by a heavy evening meal. Custom, work schedule, and personal preference seem to dictate meal patterns.

Actually, there is a wide range in eating habits, including the spacing of meals, which occurs throughout America and around the world. In primitive and poorer societies, fewer meals are consumed, with the typical pattern often being one evening meal and chance snacks throughout the day. Although these people seem to survive and reproduce, their infant mortality rates are very high, their general health is very poor, and their life span is short.

People in affluent societies are generally overfed and underactive. For somewhat different reasons, their health and life span are also very suboptimal. Many overweight and underactive people snack throughout the day, have a couple of drinks before dinner, and then eat large quantities of very rich and fatty food at the evening meal. Such a pattern has been shown to impose a severe stress on many systems of the body and, over a period of years, be a principle cause of death from heart attacks.

Research studies over the last decade have demonstrated rather convincingly that the most desirable eating habits would be those that provide an optimum amount of all nutrients to the cells at all times. This condition is achieved for the fetus via the placenta in a well-nourished woman but deteriorates throughout the life span of the child from demand feeding, to four meals a day, to three meals a day, to two and one-half meals, and sometimes to two very irregular meals a day.

Physicians have known for a long time that people fed small meals more frequently respond best to treatment. This has been the feeding schedule in first-class hospitals for many years.

Consequently, there is general agreement today that the ideal meal pattern is frequent, smaller meals, each of which provides a mixture of all the nutrients. With a little planning this can be achieved without a heavy burden being imposed on the cook and without overeating. Such a pattern provides for vitality throughout the day rather than the hungry, over-fed, drowsy, hungry sequences associated with large infrequent meals.

NUTRITION CONSULTATION

Q. *Which professionals are trained to give reliable advice about nutrition?*

A. It should be clearly understood from a legal point of view that anyone can call himself a nutritionist and give nutritional advice. There are no legal requirements. Degrees, however, are one indication of special study and preparation. The meanings of the following initials are worth remembering.

Ph.D. stands for doctor of philosophy. It is generally a research degree with specialization in a limited area of knowledge. A Ph.D. in food and nutrition from a major university is considered by most authorities to be an important prerequisite for being called a nutritionist. Such people can be found by phoning the nutrition department of a nearby college or university.

R.D. means registered dietician. The dietician has a baccalaureate degree, has successfully completed the examination for professional registration, and maintains continuing education requirements. Most R.D.s supervise food service in hospitals and other institutions and are happy to provide nutritional advice.

M.D. is doctor of medicine. Medical training is placing increasing emphasis on human nutrition. Physicians generally know what types of diets are needed when people are ill. A doctor who is not knowledgeable in nutrition will usually refer an individual to a Ph.D. in nutrition or to a registered dietitian.

Although people with advanced degrees and backgrounds in nutrition do not agree on everything, there is consensus on one general point: The best nutrition advice today is that a person eat—in moderation—a balanced variety of foods. A fitness-minded individual should be cautious about giving credibility to advice or information that does not support that consensus.

Q. *Who should consult a professional for nutritional advice?*

A. The following people should consider consultation with a professional in nutrition:

- Anyone who has, or suspects, a nutrition-related medical problem such as food intolerances and allergies.
- People whose medical problems affect their nutritional needs. Examples of such medical problems are cancer, diabetes, and high blood pressure.
- Frustrated dieters who are fed up with fad diets and are committed to changing their eating habits.

- Underweight individuals who want to gain healthy pounds.
- Pregnant women and mothers with young children trying to sort out nutrition fact.
- Athletes desiring training diets.

Dr. Harold Sandstead, Director of the Grand Forks Human Nutrition Research Center, says: "There's no free lunch in the field of nutrition. People who expect miracles or easy answers will only get ripped off. Changing poor eating and exercise habits takes commitment and time."

EATING BEFORE EXERCISE

Q. *Why should an individual refrain from eating just before exercise?*

A. When a person's large skeletal muscles are activated during strenuous exercise, they require a rich blood supply that provides nutrients and removes waste products. To do this the blood supply to the stomach and intestinal tract is reduced as the blood is mobilized to the working muscles. If food is in the stomach at this time, vomiting may result. It is best not to have eaten a meal within the previous two hours.

EXERCISE AND NAUTILUS

Q. *Exercise has been illustrated and described in so many ways. How is exercise defined?*

A. The dictionary defines exercise as ". . . exertion of the muscles to maintain bodily health."

Exercise, however, is better defined as "movement against resistance." Without resistance, there is no effective exercise. For the body to become better conditioned, the muscles have to become stronger. Muscles will not become stronger unless they are taxed with an overload. Once they are overloaded, a chemical reaction takes place within the body that causes the muscles to become stronger and better proportioned.

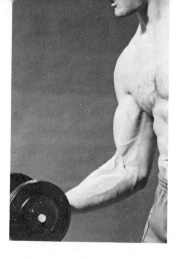

The quality of the resistance and the quantity of the movement determine the value of the exercise.

The quality of the overload or resistance determines the value of the exercise.

According to the laws of physics, everything we do involves movement that is met by some kind of resistance. Running provides resistance. Swimming provides resistance. Jumping provides resistance. Any type of muscle-powered movement is met by some kind of resistance—air, water, gravity, or friction. Exercises using an individual's body weight against air, water, or gravity, however, are not very effective ways to overload the muscles. After a short time it becomes increasingly difficult to make such movements progressively more taxing.

Adding progressive resistance to the arms, legs, torso, and other parts of the body offers a much more efficient way to overload the muscles. This type of exercise has been employed in the United States for more than fifty years. It is called weight training.

Weight training generally uses adjustable metal discs or weights that are loaded onto bars. The long bars are called barbells, and the short ones are dumbbells. Recently, weight training has become more complex, with the addition of many types of sophisticated machines. Nautilus is the best known of these machines.

Nautilus training can produce physical fitness and body-shaping results impossible to obtain in any other way. This is true only because Nautilus machines provide superior movement and superior resistance. Nautilus supplies resistance where it is needed to the degree it is needed.

Nautilus is a much more efficient form of exercise than running, swimming, lifting barbells, performing calisthenics, or doing other activities. It is the only form of exercise that is tailored to the requirements and limitations of the body itself.

RUNNING VS. NAUTILUS

Q. *Is running the best overall exercise?*

A. No. Nautilus training is much better. Nautilus can provide complete conditioning. Running is a limited midrange activity involving the large muscles of the lower half of the body. Although running can develop high levels of heart-lung endurance, it can actually reduce overall levels of muscular strength and flexibility. Running can also cause joint damage from excessive jarring every time the individual's foot hits the ground.

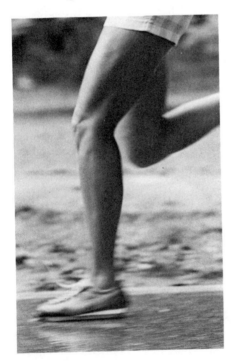

Running, rather than being one of the best overall activities for fitness, is actually one of the poorest. It decreases muscular strength and flexibility and may cause damage to the hip, knee, and ankle joints.

WEIGHT LIFTING VS. NAUTILUS TRAINING

Q. *What is the difference between weight lifting and Nautilus training?*

A. Weight lifting is a competitive sport. The goal of weight lifting is to raise as much weight on a barbell as possible while maintaining a certain form. Weight lifting not only requires strength but great skill. Anyone who has watched the "Superstars" competition on television can testify to that. Many big strong athletes perform poorly in weight lifting competition because they lack the skill to lift a heavy barbell over their heads.

Few people know that weight lifting is probably the most dangerous sport in existence today. Lifting, or a better word would be throwing, a heavy weight suddenly can easily damage the tendons, ligaments, and muscles that surround all the major joints. Most people should never attempt weight lifting.

Nautilus training, however, is a very effective activity for developing the body. It is not competitive, nor does it have the same goal as weight lifting. Its purpose is the strengthening and conditioning of the body. Instead of a one-time, sudden exertion, an individual lifts the weight slowly and smoothly 8 to 12 times. Perfect form and the correct number of repetitions are what really count.

Training on Nautilus equipment develops balanced strength and flexibility in all major muscles of the body. Furthermore, if the trainee rests no longer than fifteen seconds between machines, he can build a high level of heart-lung endurance.

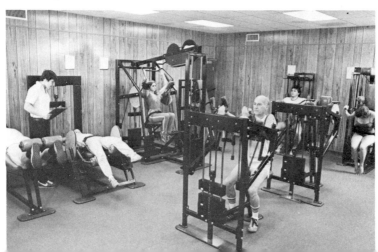

2

talking nutrition basics

NUTRIENT CLASSIFICATION

Q. *How are nutrients classified?*

A. Food is composed of various chemical compounds called nutrients. Nutrients are necessary for the proper functioning of the body and must be provided to every cell and tissue. At least fifty nutrients can be classified in the following groups according to their similarity of chemical structure or function:

1. Carbohydrates
2. Fats
3. Proteins
4. Vitamins
5. Minerals
6. Water

By far, the most abundant nutrients in foods are carbohydrates, fats, proteins, and water. Almost all of the total weight of foods is composed of these four nutrients. Vitamins and minerals occur in much smaller quantities, yet they are equally important for the proper operation of all cells. The six classes of nutrients serve the body in three general ways: (1) to provide energy for activities and heat to maintain body temperatures, (2) to provide for growth and maintenance, and (3) to control and coordinate the internal processes. All nutrients serve the body in one or more of these capacities or functions.

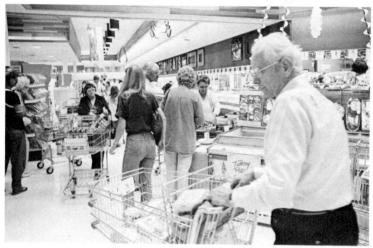

In the United States there are more than 250,000 retail food stores and the average supermarket stocks about 11,000 items. Never before in our history has the food supply been of such quantity as well as quality.

Few foods are pure carbohydrate, protein, or fat. Table syrups and sugar are all carbohydrate. Cooking oils are all fat. Plain, unflavored gelatin is nearly all protein. Almost all other food is made up of a mixture of nutrients.

ESSENTIAL AND NONESSENTIAL NUTRIENTS

Q. *Which nutrients are essential and which are nonessential?*

A. An essential nutrient is one that cannot be synthesized from simpler materials ordinarily present in the diet at a sufficient rate for optimum health. Essential nutrients must be supplied in the diet. Nonessential nutrients are also needed by the cells but can be synthesized in the body from simpler materials provided in the diet or from the breakdown of other cell components. For the most efficient operation of cell metabolism and body function, both essential and nonessential nutrients should be present in the diet.

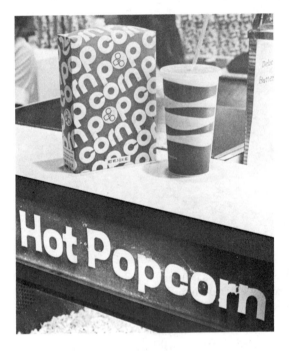

Food is a part of almost every social function, but customs vary. Popcorn is a part of going to the movies but is unacceptable at the opera.

Essential Nutrients (must be present in the diet)

1. Sources of energy: carbohydrates or fats
2. Polyunsaturated fatty acid or linoleic acid
3. Threonine
4. Tryptophan
5. Lysine
6. Leucine
7. Iso-leucine
8. Methionine

9. Valine
10. Phenylalanine
11. Histidine (may be essential for infants)
12. Arginine (may be essential for adults)
13. Vitamin A
14. Vitamin D
15. Vitamin E
16. Vitamin K
17. Ascorbic acid (vitamin C)
18. Thiamin
19. Riboflavin
20. Niacin
21. Pyridoxine
22. Folic acid
23. Pantothenic acid
24. Biotin
25. Vitamin B_{12}
26. Calcium
27. Phosphorus
28. Sodium
29. Chloride
30. Potassium
31. Magnesium
32. Iron
33. Copper
34. Manganese
35. Iodine
36. Cobalt
37. Zinc
38. Fluoride
39. Molybdenum
40. Selenium
41. Chromium
42. Water

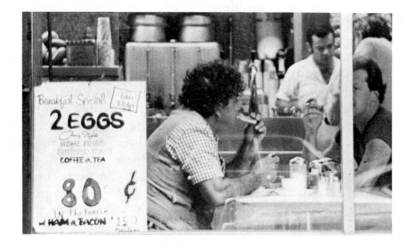

The directive to eat breakfast is good advice for all people.

Some of the Nonessential Nutrients (required by the cells)

1. Carbohydrates
2. Fats
3. Choline
4. Glycine
5. Alanine
6. Cysteine
7. Cystine
8. Serine
9. Tyrosine
10. Aspartic acid
11. Glutamic acid
12. Proline
13. Hydroxyproline

Many other compounds are required by the body for its normal function or operation. These compounds can be made by the cells from the end products of metabolism or from other nutrients present in the diet. Although the nonessential nutrients can be made in the body, it would prefer to ingest them. A diet that includes the essential and nonessential nutrients would provide for the most efficient operation of the cells.

TASTE SENSATIONS

Q. *Do taste sensations change as a person ages?*

A. Taste changes considerably with age. Flavors are recognized by small structures in the tongue called taste buds. An average person's taste buds number about 10,000. They respond to four different flavors. Those at the tip of the tongue register sweetness; those at the sides, sourness; those at the back, bitterness; and all of them respond to saltiness.

Children have more taste buds than adults. The young tend to prefer sweetness, partly because of their larger number of responsive buds and partly because their energy requirements need replenishment more often than adults.

In adulthood, however, the bitterness taste buds seem to become dominant. This accounts for some people's preference for bitter-tasting alcoholic beverages and foods. But as most people reach later life, their tip-of-the-tongue taste buds become less sensitive. At age 70, they may desire more sweetness in their food than they did at age 40.

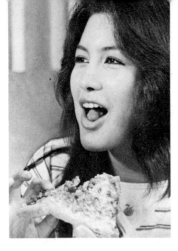

The many flavors from foods are recognized by thousands of taste buds located on the surface of the tongue.

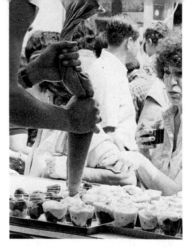

People of all races and cultures have a natural, inborn preference for sweet-tasting foods.

Q. *Do certain foods taste different to women than to men?*
A. Yes; there seems to be a link between taste sensitivity and female hormone levels. When these hormone levels change dramatically, as in pregnancy, taste can vary accordingly. This is part of the reason that pregnant women get cravings for some foods, especially those that are sour.

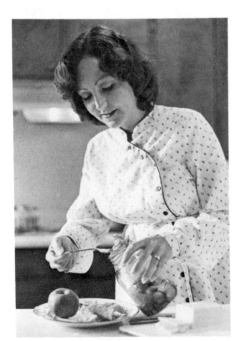

Pregnant women often get cravings for particular foods such as sour pickles. These cravings are usually related to changes in hormone levels.

DIGESTION

Q. *How are foods digested?*

A. The digestive tract is composed of the mouth, esophagus, stomach, small intestine, and large intestine. The mechanical and chemical phases of digestion occur in these organs. The mechanical phase of digestion is responsible for the subdividing, mixing, and propelling of the food mass along the digestive tract. It includes chewing, swallowing, and the muscular activity of the walls of the digestive tract itself. The chemical phase of digestion, which is responsible for the final breakdown of food particles, is brought about by the digestive enzymes. Enzymes act as catalysts in the body. They increase the rate of a reaction without becoming part of the final reaction product. Digestive enzymes aid in the breakdown of large nutrient molecules into smaller molecules. For example, carbohydrates are changed into simple sugars, fats into glycerol and fatty acids, and proteins into amino acids.

The process of digestion starts when food enters the body through the mouth where it is chewed, broken into small pieces, and mixed with saliva. The fluid secreted by the salivary glands contains digestive enzymes that act upon carbohydrates. From the mouth, the food passes to the stomach by way of the esophagus. The digestion of certain foods continues in the stomach under the influence of the secretions and churning action of the stomach wall. Ordinarily, a mixed meal leaves the stomach in three or four hours. This time can vary, however, according to the composition of the diet. Carbohydrates leave the stomach most rapidly, followed by proteins. Fats remain in the stomach for the longest period of time. Thus, the sensation of hunger will occur sooner after a meal that is relatively high in carbohydrate than after a meal containing adequate amounts of protein or fat.

After leaving the stomach, the liquified food mass, called chyme, passes into the small intestine for further absorption into the body. The small intestine is affected by secretions from its walls and from the liver and pancreas. The undi-

THE DIGESTIVE TRACT

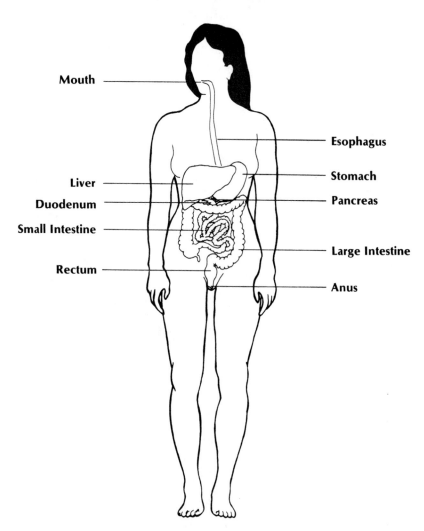

Mouth

Esophagus

Stomach

Liver

Pancreas

Duodenum

Small Intestine

Large Intestine

Rectum

Anus

Food passes via the mouth and throat to the stomach, where it becomes a
semiliquid pulp known as chyme. This is gradually squeezed into the small
intestine, where nearly all digestion and absorption take place. Most of
the water is absorbed into the bloodstream from the large intestine, from
which food residue is passed to the rectum and excreted.

gested food residues pass from the small intestine into the large intestine or colon. This material also contains some of the end products of digestion such as water, as well as waste materials. These waste products travel through the large intestine and are stored in the rectum where they await periodic excretion from the body.

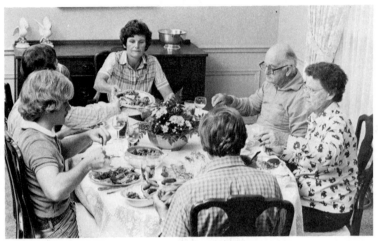

Food plays a central part in people's beliefs about life. Joy is celebrated in feasts—whether they be an American Thanksgiving dinner, a European country wedding, or a tribal celebration—and special, more expensive foods may be prepared. Ritual overeating may be practiced at such times.

Q. *What makes a person's stomach growl and rumble?*

A. The stomach and intestines are active parts of the digestive process. The stomach churns food and the intestines squeeze it along the alimentary canal. As a result of this activity, slurping and rumbling noises are produced. Usually a person cannot hear them without a stethoscope. But sometimes the sound is extra loud. This can occur when a great deal of air is in the stomach with certain foods or when the stomach contains no food but expects it.

Q. *Since the stomach contains many strong acids, why doesn't it digest itself?*

A. The strongest stomach acid is hydrochloric. It can actually burn holes in a wooden floor. The reason hydrochloric acid does not burn holes in the stomach itself is the stomach's special lining, which produces a thick protective mucus. This coating allows food to be attacked by strong acids but keeps them away from the stomach walls.

ABSORPTION

Q. *What happens after foods are digested?*
A. Absorption follows digestion. The function of digestion, in fact, is to prepare the nutrients for absorption through the walls of the digestive tract. Most of this absorption takes place in the small intestine, although water and small amounts of simple sugars and alcohol pass through the mucosa of the stomach into the bloodstream, while various minerals and water are absorbed in the large intestine. Fingerlike projections on the wall of the intestines into the food canal, called *villi,* increase the absorptive surface area about 600-fold.

CIRCULATION AND RESPIRATION

Q. *Is the process complete after digestion and absorption?*
A. No, other processes such as circulation, respiration, and metabolism are equally important.

Each villus contains a network of tiny vessels that drink up the nutrients as they pass along the food canal. Actually, there are two kinds of tiny vessels in each villus: one that contains lymph and accepts digested fats (lymphatic vessels) and one that contains blood and accepts all other digested nutrients (capillaries). These little vessels are the means by which the absorbed nutrients are circulated to every cell throughout the body.

The lungs are the route of entry for another very important cell nutrient: oxygen. Analogous to the villi in the intestines are the alveoli in the lungs. These are tiny projections into the air canal. Like the intestinal villi, alveoli contain a network of tiny vessels that contain blood and drink up the oxygen as it is inhaled into the lungs.

Nutrients then circulate throughout the body in a manner analogous to diners at a cafeteria. As the blood flows by, cells take what they need. Excess nutrients may be stored, converted to more complex compounds, or excreted.

Food, as consumed, is of no use to the body. It must first be broken down into smaller pieces so it can be swallowed, and then digested into smaller molecules so it can be absorbed to feed the cells.

For example, a carrot contains several vitamins, some starch that is a form of carbohydrate, some poor-quality protein, several minerals, and water. Once the carrot has been digested and its nutrients are absorbed and transported to the cells, they are accepted according to need and function of that particular cell. Its vitamin A would be accepted for use in the retina of the eye and various other cells throughout the body or picked up by the liver for storage. The starch digested to glucose would be picked up to be used as an energy source by any cell in the body or stored in the liver or

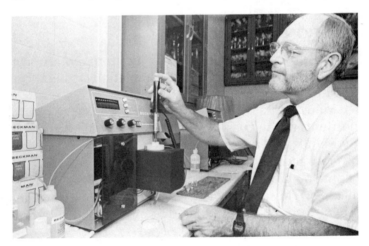

Dr. Robert Cade, Professor of Medicine at the University of Florida's College of Medicine, has been deeply involved in research on the circulation and metabolism of nutrients in the human body. Over the past 20 years, Dr. Cade has worked with many football players and marathon runners.

muscle as glycogen. Or, if the glycogen stores were filled, it would be picked up by the fat storage cells where it is converted to and stored as fat. The protein digested to amino acids would be used or converted to glycogen or fat for storage. The minerals would be picked up for use and the extra amounts would either be accepted by cells or excreted by the kidneys in the urine.

CONSTIPATION

Q. *What causes constipation?*

A. The word *constipation* means simply "delay in the passage of stool." Delay, however, tends to be interpreted in many ways. Some people say they are constipated when they do not have a bowel action every day at the same time. Other people believe they are constipated unless their stools pass without making expulsive effort. Yet others relate constipation to a feeling of bloat or uneasiness in the gut.

None of these beliefs is accurate. True constipation can only be diagnosed in the context of what is normal for an individual. Surveys have shown that the range of normal varies from two bowel movements a week to three a day. As long as a person is functioning normally in every other way, then whatever is normal for him is normal.

Diet obviously plays an important role in constipation. Stools are made up of undigested food waste, dead bacteria, secretions from the intestines, and water. During digestion, water is constantly being extracted from the material inside the gut and passed back into the body's general supply. It takes four to six hours for the food that enters the stomach to be pushed out into the small intestine, in a liquid state. It spends five hours in the small intestines, still very moist, and up to 24 hours in the large intestines, where it becomes progressively drier. The longer the food material spends in the large intestines, the more it is going to dry out. Hard, dry stools are painful to pass and can lead to true constipation.

An individual can assist the passage of stools from his body by making certain that ample amounts of fruits, vegetables, grains, and liquids are consumed on a daily basis.

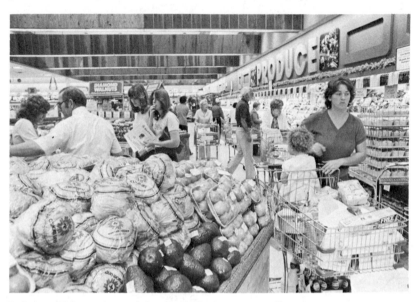

Eating a wide variety of foods each day, especially adequate amounts of fruits and vegetables, assists the body in the evacuation process.

METABOLISM

Q. *What is metabolism?*

A. Metabolism is a term used to describe all the chemical changes that occur in the body.

Once the cell accepts a nutrient, it is carried to certain parts of the cell where it enters into various chemical reactions. In general, these reactions are either constructive (anabolic) or destructive (catabolic). The constructive reactions are associated with growth, pregnancy, lactation, and healing. The destructive reactions are associated with the release of energy when nutrients are burned or broken down during infections, during muscle wasting, and during the continuous destruction of worn-out cells. Both processes go on simultaneously in different parts or cells of the body.

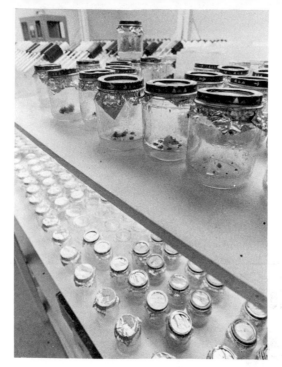

Approximately 10,000 research papers are reported each year in the world's literature on food and nutrition. One ongoing study at the University of Florida involves producing embryos from vegetative tissues, such as pecan, peach, orange, apple, and avocado. This photograph shows bottles and test tubes of identical clones, which will be researched carefully under various growing conditions.

Each cell in the body can be considered a microscopic part of the whole organism. It must receive a source of energy, oxygen, vitamins, amino acids, and minerals for use in making enzymes and the other necessary cell components that are needed to maintain the cell and carry out the functions assigned to it. Each cell must be protected and kept warm; it must be able to rid itself of its waste products; and it must be sensitive and able to react to various stimuli. It is born, matures, lives for a while, dies, and is broken down. Certain parts are reused, and the rest are carried off for excretion.

In short, the human body is the most complex machine on earth. Man has never been able to create a machine that is comparable to his body or to understand completely the complex interaction of all these components in building, maintaining, and regulating the body processes.

3

estimating caloric needs

ENERGY AND THE SUN

Q. *What is energy and where does it come from?*

A. Energy is the internal power an individual must have for everything he does. Breathing, sleeping, digesting, even expressing joy or anger, require energy.

The sun is the ultimate source of energy. In high school biology, students learn that energy cannot be created or destroyed. It can only change its form and the place where it is available.

Only plants have the ability to grow by combining the energy from the sun with the elements from the air, soil, and water. Animals usually get their energy from plants. Humans get energy from plants and animals. From a nutritional viewpoint, food and energy are measured in *calories*.

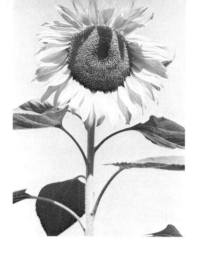

This sunflower symbolizes the fact that the energy of life comes from one source—the sun. Humans have no way to take in this energy directly, but plants can trap solar energy by using it to combine carbon dioxide and water. The product of this combination is a hydrated carbon, or carbohydrate. (Photo by Ellington Darden)

CALORIE DEFINED

Q. *What is a calorie?*

A. Energy from food as well as activity is typically measured as heat and expressed as calories. A calorie (kilo-calorie is actually the more appropriate term) is the amount of heat it takes to raise the temperature of one liter of water one degree centigrade. To help a person visualize this fact, 100 calories would raise the temperature of one liter (approximately one quart) of water from freezing level to boiling. A calorie, therefore, is not a nutrient but a unit of measure. It is used to express the energy value of foods or the energy required by the body to perform a given task.

ENERGY VALUES OF FOOD

Q. *How are the energy values of food determined?*

A. The energy values of foods are established by measuring the calories of heat given off when the food is burned in equipment specially designed for the purpose. The bomb calorimeter is the most widely used instrument to measure the energy value of food. A weighed sample of food is placed in the bomb, which is filled with oxygen. This container is then placed in an insulated water bath that contains a known amount of water. The food in the bomb is burned completely after an electric spark ignites the food. The heat given off causes the temperature of the bomb and then the surrounding water to increase a certain number of degrees per gram of that particular food. A sensitive thermometer, which can be read to a thousandth of a degree, is used to measure the temperature of the water before and after combustion. From the increase in the temperature reading, the energy value or fuel value of the food can be calculated.

The bomb calorimeter was originally used to establish the caloric values of pure fat, carbohydrate, and protein. It was soon discovered, however, that several corrections were necessary when calculating the energy values of human diets, because the body was not as efficient as the calorimeter. Extensive experimentation revealed that the following figures were suitable for estimating the amount of energy supplied by various mixed diets:

> 1 gram of carbohydrate = 4 calories
> 1 gram of fat   = 9 calories
> 1 gram of protein   = 4 calories

CALORIE TABLES

Q. *How accurate are calorie tables?*

A. Calorie tables are carefully done and based on averages of many analyses. Even though they are estimates, they can be used with a reasonable degree of accuracy (see Appendix B).

AVERAGE SERVINGS

Q. *What is an average serving?*

A. An average serving can be defined in numerous ways. A serving of mashed potatoes is about the same size as a large scoop or one serving of ice cream. A serving of meat is usually considered to be three ounces, a serving of orange juice is about three ounces or half a cup, and a serving of apple pie is one-sixth of a nine-inch pie. In addition, a serving of egg is the whole thing, a serving of bread is one slice, and a serving of cereal is three-quarters of a cup.

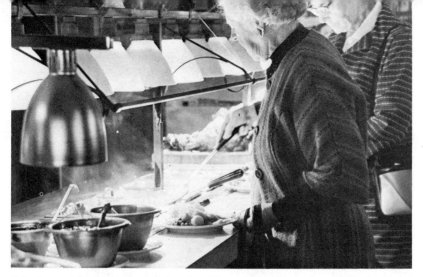

Caloric needs decrease with advancing years because metabolism and muscular activity are reduced. A 5% reduction per decade in caloric intake is a suggested guideline.

CALORIC NEEDS

Q. *What determines the caloric need of an individual?*

A. The total caloric requirement of an individual is the amount of energy required for maintaining basal metabolism, physical activity, sleep, growth, pregnancy, lactation, rehabilitation from disease or inactivity, the specific dynamic effect, and the maintenance of ideal body temperature. The basal metabolism is the minimum amount of cell reaction needed to carry on the vital or life processes of the body when it is awake. Energy required for the performance of physical activity ranks second to the amount of energy required for basal metabolism. Energy must also be supplied to meet the needs of an increasing number or increasing activity of cells during growth, pregnancy, lactation, or rehabilitation from disease or inactivity.

The extra energy required to utilize nutrients by the cells, specific dynamic effect, is the fourth factor that is part of the total energy requirement, although this factor is relatively small. Finally, an amount of energy is required to maintain the ideal body temperature if the environment is very hot or cold. Under very cold conditions, the typical inefficiency and energy loss from the cell reactions is not sufficient to maintain ideal body temperature. If a person's clothing is unable to

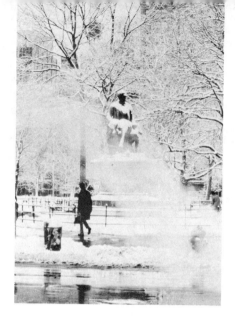

When a person becomes chilled, his body begins to shiver. Shivering causes the body to generate more heat by burning additional calories. (Photo by Jonathan Taylor)

keep the body warmth in and the cold air out, he may begin to shiver or stamp his feet in order to generate more body warmth by causing more cells to become active. Under very hot conditions, the body may actually have to work to keep cool by increasing the rate of respiration and by perspiring profusely.

BASAL METABOLISM

Q. *How can basal metabolism be determined?*

A. The basal energy requirement of an individual can be determined by a respiration apparatus. This apparatus measures the oxygen used during a specific period of time, which is dependent upon the amount of oxidation or energy utilization taking place in his body.

The energy used or required affects the subject's basal or minimal metabolism if the measurement is made while the subject is awake but completely relaxed and rested, is not under emotional stress, has fasted overnight, and if the test is conducted at a comfortable temperature and humidity. These results are expressed as calories per day and reflect the amount of energy required for maintenance of a person's minimal activities.

It is more practical for individuals to estimate their own basal energy requirement. One simple method is based on body weight as follows:

Basal Energy Requirement = 1 cal. × body weight (kg.)
                                               × 24 hrs. (in cal./24 hrs.)

The kilograms of body weight are found by dividing the weight in pounds by 2.2. The calculation for the energy needed for the basal metabolism of a college man weighing 187 pounds would be:

Basal Energy Requirement = 1 × 187/2.2 × 24
                                          = 2,040 cal./24 hrs.

The basal metabolism or energy requirement is also affected by factors other than body weight such as body composition, age, climate, sex, general health, growth, pregnancy, and lactation.

ENERGY FOR ACTIVITIES

Q. *How is the energy required for physical activities calculated?*

A. Any kind of physical activity increases the energy expenditure above the basal caloric need, even if the activity is merely eating, sitting, or standing. The amount of energy needed for physical activity by the moderately active man or woman usually comprises the second greatest caloric expenditure. This would not be true for a very active individual, such as a basketball player, a distance runner, or a lumberjack. In these subjects, the energy required for physical activity would probably exceed the basal energy requirement.

Several factors determine the energy cost of physical activity: the kind of activity, the intensity and duration of the activity performed, the skill of the participant, and the body size of the individual. The table below lists factors that can be used to calculate the cost of certain physical activities.

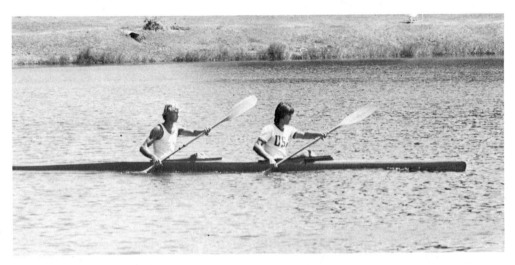

Muscular work is by far the most important factor that raises the energy requirements above the basal rate. (Photo by Inge Cook)

Estimation of Calories for Activities for Various Types of Days

Type of Activity	Cal. per lb. per hr.
A. At rest most of the day (sitting, reading, etc.; very little walking and standing)	0.23
B. Very light exercise (sitting most of the day, studying, with about 2 hrs. of walking and standing)	0.27
C. Light exercise (sitting, typing, standing, laboratory work, walking, etc.)	0.36
D. Moderate exercise (standing, walking, housework, gardening, carpentry, etc.; little sitting)	0.50
E. Severe exercise (standing, walking, skating, outdoor games, dancing, etc.; little sitting)	0.77
F. Very severe exercise (sports—tennis, swimming, basketball, football, running—heavy work, etc.; little sitting)	1.09

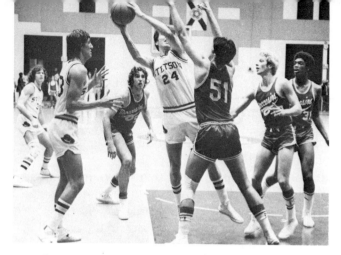

Competitive basketball, because it requires much starting, stopping, jumping, running, and changing of directions, requires a large number of calories. (Courtesy of Stetson University)

CALORIES FOR MENTAL EXERTION

Q. *How many calories are required during mental exertion?*

A. Not many. One researcher, in fact, calculated that the energy needed for one hour of hard thinking could be supplied by half a peanut. This would amount to only several calories.

In contrast to vigorous sporting activities, reading and studying require only a few calories.

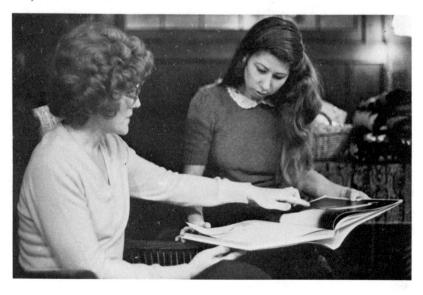

ENERGY FOR GROWTH

Q. *What about the energy required for growth, repair, pregnancy, and lactation?*

A. The energy required for growth, repair, pregnancy, and lactation changes and depends on the rate or stage of the growth process. If adequate amounts of energy sources are not provided, growth is retarded and finally all cell activity is reduced. Approximately 10% of the body's energy sources are used during growth or repair of tissues.

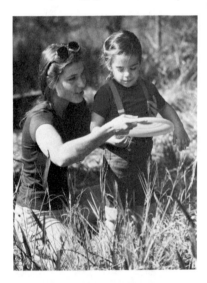

Nutrient needs of children are based on age, height, and weight. Because of their rapid growth and metabolism, children require more calories per pound than do adults. (Photo by Inge Cook)

ENERGY FOR FOOD UTILIZATION

Q. *How many calories does it take to utilize food itself?*

A. Energy required to utilize food has been referred to as a tax that is added to the total calorie intake for utilizing the ingested nutrients. If the diet was exclusively one of the following foods, the tax would be: carbohydrate—6%, fat—14%, and protein—30% of the caloric value of that food. Since most people eat a mixed diet, the average energy increase is estimated to be less than 10%. By adding together the calories for basal metabolism and physical activities and taking 10% of this total, the energy required to digest, absorb, and metabolize food can be estimated. In this way the total amount of

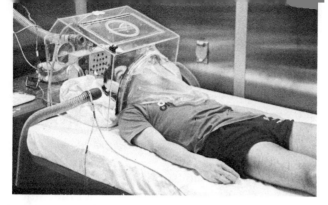

Research concerning the specific dynamic action of food was being carried out at Pennsylvania State University when this photograph was taken in April of 1981. A subject fasts for 12 hours and is fed a 1,000-calorie liquid meal. He is then placed in an experimental rest chamber for three hours. As the subject rests, his body temperature, heart rate, and energy metabolism are monitored. (Photo by Ellington Darden)

energy required by an individual can be determined. The table below shows an example of such combined estimates.

Shortcut Method of Estimating Daily Calorie Need

A. Weigh yourself: using your body weight as a basis, estimate your basal calorie need for twenty-four hours.

B. Keep a diary of your activities for a typical day. Decide from the table on page 50 in which category you belong: A, B, C, D, E, or F. Calculate the calorie need for your activities for one day.

C. Total your calorie needs, taking into consideration the 10-percent "tax" for utilization of food.
Sample of calculation:
Assume: an adult weighing 125 lbs. (57 kg.)
a day with 16 hrs. of activity: 8 hrs. of sleep
category of activity: C, light exercise

1. Calories for basal metabolism (corrected for saving in sleep):
Basal metabolism for 24 hrs.: 1,368 cal. (1 x 57 x 24)
Saving in sleep, 8 hrs.: $\underline{-46}$ cal. (0.1 x 57 x 8)
1,322

2. Add calories for activity (0.36 x 125 x 16) = 720;
1,322 + 720 = 2,042

3. Add calories for the influence of food (10% of 2,042) = 204

4. Total estimated calories needed for the day (2,042 + 204)
= 2,246

CALORIES BURNED FROM NAUTILUS WORKOUT

Q. How many calories does an average individual burn during a Nautilus workout?

A. The answer to this question depends on age, sex, body composition, the resistance on each machine, and several other factors. Some general guidelines, however, should be considered.

Walking briskly requires about 5 calories per minute, bicycling consumes 8 calories per minute, jogging burns up 10 calories per minute, and swimming uses up 11 calories per minute. Since walking, bicycling, jogging, and swimming are basically midrange activities, they would require fewer calories per minute than full-range exercise on Nautilus equipment. Exercise properly performed on Nautilus equipment would require between 15 and 20 calories per minute. The machines that involve the largest muscle groups would burn the most calories.

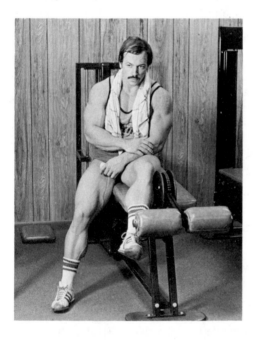

The average individual who trains on Nautilus equipment would burn between 15 and 20 calories per minute per machine. Athletes, who are bigger and stronger than the average person, would burn more calories. (Photo by Inge Cook)

For example, let us assume that a 175-pound, 30-year-old man performs a standard Nautilus workout. He does twelve exercises, five for his lower body and seven for his upper body. Let us also assume that each exercise takes one minute to perform.

To estimate the calories he burns for this workout, we can multiply the five lower body exercises by 20 and the seven upper body exercises by 15. Thus, 5 × 20 = 100, and 7 × 15 = 105, or 205 calories total. This total would increase as the resistance and repetitions progress.

Sports with Small Energy Costs. Many sports are single efforts, such as the shot put, discus, diving, and ski jumping. Others are of short duration, such as short-distance skiing and swimming, sprinting, and hurdling. Although these events require strength and ability to react quickly, the energy needs are increased relatively little if these sports are practiced less than an hour a day. Additional sports that require relatively small amounts of energy expenditure are listed below:

Archery
Baseball
Boating
Bowling
Canoeing, slow or moderate
    speed
Cycling, slow or moderate
    speed
Dancing
Diving
Equestrian sports
Fencing
Golf
Softball
Tennis

High jump
Hurdle races
Javelin throw
Pole vaulting
Rowing, slow or moderate
    speed
Shooting
Short-distance running
Short-distance skiing
Short-distance swimming
Shot put
Skating
Ski jumping
Volleyball
Weight lifting

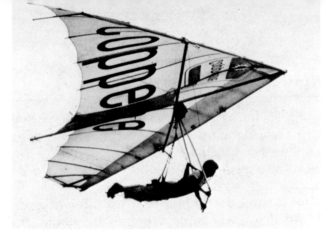

Hang-gliding is basically a low-energy sport.

Sports with Large Energy Costs. Sports requiring extra energy expenditure over long periods of time are listed here. Preseason conditioning and the hours of training required for sports such as swimming, track, football, and basketball may increase the total caloric needs to as high as 4,000 to 5,000 calories per day, depending on body size and weight. A list of sports that require relatively large amounts of any expenditure follows:

Basketball
Boxing
Football
Gymnastics (especially apparatus)
Handball
Hockey (ice and field)
Judo
Long-distance canoeing
Long-distance rowing
Long-distance running
Long-distance skating
Long-distance skiing
Long-distance swimming
Marathon
Middle-distance running
Mountaineering
Paddleball
Pentathlon
Skin diving
Squash
Soccer
Tumbling
Water polo
Wrestling

Almost any sport with relatively low energy cost can be placed in the high-energy classification if it is carried on intensively for a long time. For example, the prolonged golf game or tennis match could also fall into this category.

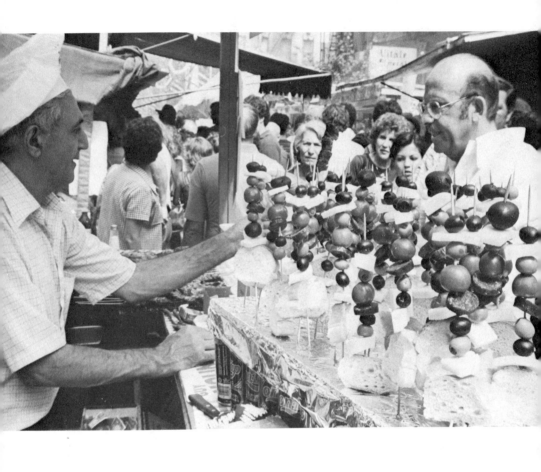

II.

NUTRIENTS

4

proteins

IMPORTANCE OF PROTEIN

Q. *What are proteins?*

A. Proteins are simply large molecules built from amino acids. Half of the dry matter of an adult is protein. Of this amount one-third is in the form of muscle, one-third in bone and cartilage, one-tenth in the skin, and the rest in other tissues and in body fluids. Because these tissues regularly need additional proteins for maintenance, the body must have a regular supply of protein in the diet.

In order for the body to use protein, food must be broken down into amino acids in the digestive tract. The amino acids are absorbed by the body and then resynthesized into proteins necessary for the body. The body requires a vast number of proteins, but they are all formed from the same pool of amino acids.

PROTEIN FOODS

Q. *What are protein foods?*

A. When we eat a source of protein, chemicals in the stomach act on the protein to liberate the amino acids. Thus, protein foods are foods that contain appreciable amounts of amino acids. Meat, dairy products, chicken, and fish are examples of protein foods.

There is also another type of commercially prepared protein food. These are the popular protein supplements, which include protein pills, liquids, and powders. They are made from such things as skimmed milk powder, powdered liver, yeast, egg whites, beef organs, calcium caseinate, and soybeans. Most brands carry wording on the label that is similar to "Super Protein" or "High-Protein" and contain high percentages of protein with very small amounts of fat and carbohydrate. They are, however, rather expensive at $7.95 or more a pound. When sufficient protein is obtained through regular good eating habits, such supplements are not necessary.

PROTEIN QUALITY

Q. *What about protein quality? Are some protein foods better than others?*

A. In order to select adequate sources of dietary protein, it is important to understand the concept of protein quality. Proteins may be classified simply in two categories: high-quality or complete proteins and poor-quality or incomplete proteins. The high-quality protein has an amino acid composition closer to that of animal tissues and human requirements than a poor-quality protein. Body or tissue proteins are composed of amino acids; the body cannot synthesize some of these foods. These must be provided in the diet. The food, consequently, that has the greatest amount of these essential amino acids present in it has the highest biological value.

The original source of proteins is plants. Animals cannot "fix" nitrogen in their tissues as can plants. They must obtain their proteins or nitrogenous compounds from plants or other animals that have consumed plants. Proteins from plant and animal tissue are not of the same quality because they do not contain the same amount or the same kinds of amino acids. It turns out that the food items that supply the highest-quality proteins for humans come from animal tissues like beef, pork, fish, chicken, eggs, and dairy products. It should not be surprising that the composition of animal tissues is more similar to that of human tissues than is the composition of plant tissues. After all, we are more like cows than carrots.

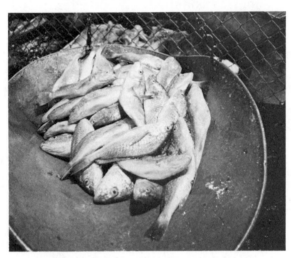

Fish is an excellent source of high-quality protein.

DAILY PROTEIN REQUIREMENTS

Q. *How much protein is needed each day?*

A. Protein is measured in grams. The gram is a basic unit in the metric system that equals about $\frac{1}{28}$ of an ounce. There are 454 grams in a pound. Food composition tables list protein in grams. For example: eight ounces of milk contain nine grams of protein, a large egg has six grams, and a six-ounce steak has 48 grams. A person should examine food composition tables for complete listings.

Nutritionists have devised a simple rule of thumb to determine adequate protein levels for athletes. They recommend

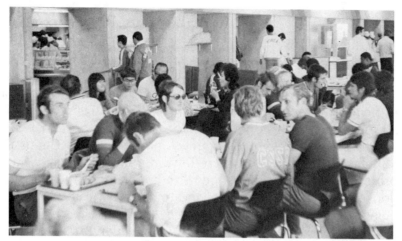

A survey taken at the Olympic Village cafeteria in Montreal revealed that the typical athlete consumed a daily average of about 5,500 calories. This survey also showed that most of these calories came from 2.4 pounds of meat—hardly a diet lacking in protein! (Photo by Ellington Darden)

0.8 grams of protein daily for each kilogram of body weight. Or, stated another way, *.36 grams of protein are needed for each pound a person weighs.* An individual can determine his need by multiplying his weight in pounds by .36.

The table below shows calculations for some weights. The requirements are essentially the same for men and women.

Bodyweight (in pounds)	Daily Protein (in grams)
100	36
112	40
125	45
137	49
150	54
167	60
175	63
187	67
200	72
212	76
225	81

Q. *How is the Recommended Dietary Allowance for protein determined?*

A. According to Dr. Mark Hegsted, administrator of the Agriculture Department's Human Nutrition Center: "There are, in general, three methods for estimating protein needs and these have been used in developing the RDA. The first is to measure the nitrogen excretion when individuals are fed a protein-free diet. The nitrogen excretion under these conditions provides an estimate of the total body protein which is being broken down and would have to be replaced by dietary protein. The second is to measure nitrogen balance when different levels of protein are fed. In a normal adult, who does not need to form additional tissue but only has to maintain his body composition, the total intake and the total excretion should be the same. Thus, the minimal intake which will permit nitrogen balance is a measure of requirements. Finally, there is a lot of information about what people eat and their state of health in general. If health is generally maintained, one has to assume that protein intakes are adequate.

"The RDA are derived, therefore, by looking at the data obtained from the first two methods, which provide estimates

One of the standard tests that scientists use to measure the protein needs of the body is the Kjeldahl method for determining nitrogen. Nitrogen balance studies reveal that each day the vast majority of Americans consume more than twice as much protein than they actually require for optimum fitness.

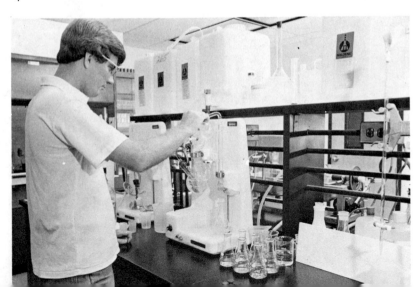

of the minimal need, and than adding corrections to account for differences in individuals and different diets. The RDA have always been set higher that the estimates of minimal need. Finally, these data are compared to what we know about dietary habits in general. If such estimates resulted in values that were clearly out of line with what healthy people eat, they would certainly be suspect. The RDA then are estimates based on all of the information available. It should be emphasized that they are deliberately set substantially above the estimates of minimal need so that we have no reason to believe that individuals who consume these amounts will not receive enough. People may consume less and be well fed."

To determine the RDA for protein, the scientist starts with the reference man and the bell-shaped curve. The reference man weighs 70 kilograms. The bell-shaped curve has equal segments on either side of the mean. These segments are spoken of as standard deviations. One standard deviation would be approximately plus or minus about 66% of the population. Two standard deviations cover 98% of the population.

The total nitrogen requirements for the reference man when they are transformed to protein amount to 23.8 grams daily. This means that 50% of the population will have their requirements satisfied by 23.8 grams or less of protein per day. And 98% of the population would have their protein needs met by 30.8 grams of protein per day.

Since people do not consume ideal measures of amino acids at each meal, another 30% increment was added to the figure. Now the protein requirements per day is 40 grams, which is .57 grams per kilogram of body weight. This is a safe level for protein of good biological value.

Just to be doubly sure that there was no question about the rationale, the figure was boosted from .57 grams per kilogram of body weight to .8. Thus, the Food and Nutrition Board's final figure of daily protein for the reference man amounts to .8 times 70 kilograms of body weight, or 56 grams.

The RDA for protein, 56 grams for the reference man, is really a high figure. For 98% of the population, it is twice as much as they actually need.

MASSIVE AMOUNTS OF PROTEIN

Q. *Should large amounts of protein foods and protein supplements be considered an essential part of the diet of an athlete or an individual on a Nautilus training program?*

A. Contrary to what many people believe, and contrary to what physical fitness and health magazines would have their readers believe, Americans get more than enough protein. This is especially true of athletes and other fitness-minded people. Surveys show that most athletes consume four to five times their actual protein requirements each day. There are absolutely *no* health or performance benefits from excessive high-protein eating.

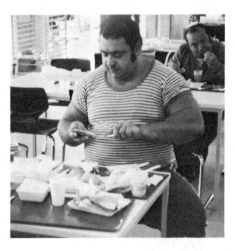

Vasily Alexeev, 345-pound Russian weight lifter and holder of many world records, was eating lunch at the Olympic Village cafeteria in Munich when this photograph was taken. It is not unusual for Alexeev to consume 1,500 grams of protein daily—more than 10 times his actual requirements! In all probability, he has excessive growth of his liver and kidneys. (Photo by Ellington Darden)

Q. *Why do athletes believe that massive amounts of protein are necessary during intensive training?*

A. This belief probably evolved from the ancient Olympic Games. These athletes thought they obtained strength from eating raw meat of animals, such as lions and tigers, that displayed great fighting strength. Although few athletes today consume raw meat, the idea that "you are what you eat" still exists.

During the early 1900s, scientists began to unravel some of the mysteries behind muscle physiology. They found that muscles are primarily composed of water, lipids, and proteins. Wrongly, athletes and coaches began to believe that "muscles are made of protein." What the scientists said, however, was that muscles are 70% water, 22% protein, and 7% lipids. Only if a muscle is devoid of water is it mostly protein. But athletes and coaches never bothered to study all the data. They wanted to believe that muscles were made of protein because this justified their centuries-old meat-eating practices.

The protein beliefs of athletes and coaches were further reinforced in the later 1930s by some magazine publishers. The first protein supplements were advertised and sold in these magazines devoted to fitness and bodybuilding. The advertisements tried to convince the reader that the most efficient way to get protein would be through the advertised supplements. It was claimed in the advertisement that "protein supplements build muscle, strength, and health." All these concepts were misleading then and are misleading today.

PROTEIN SUPPLEMENTS

Q. *How big is the protein supplement business in the United States?*

A. In 1974 approximately 40 companies manufactured protein supplements with an estimated annual sales volume of $70 million. The business was dominated by fewer than 10 companies whose products accounted for 80% of all sales.

Growth of the protein supplement industry has paralleled the increasing interest in health foods. During 1980 the health food industry expected to gross $3 billion.

Many of the buyers of protein supplements have seen the advertisements for these products in health and fitness magazines. Not surprisingly, as noted in the preceding question, protein supplement users consider these magazines reliable sources of nutritional information. For many other protein supplement users, however, the label they see on the item in the store is their only source of such information.

The Federal Trade Commission's January 15, 1979, staff report on the *Advertising and Labeling of Protein Supplements* deals in detail with the controversial consumer attitudes regarding the supplements.

PROTEIN SUPPLEMENT RIP-OFF

Q. *Specifically, what did the Federal Trade Commission find in its investigation of the protein supplement industry?*

A. The following 10 conclusions summarize the findings of the Federal Trade Commission regarding advertising and labeling of protein supplements:

1. The use of concentrated protein supplements without medical supervision poses risks to the health of infants, young children, and persons with liver or kidney disorders.

2. The level of protein concentration at which substantial health risks arise is usually from 20–40% of the calories ingested.

3. The Recommended Dietary Allowance for protein is a sufficiently reliable index of the protein requirements of 97.5% of all healthy Americans.

4. No large percentage of Americans fails to consume adequate amounts of protein.

5. There are no significant nutritional benefits from the use of protein supplements.

6. Protein is not depleted in any greater degree through strenuous activity than through ordinary physical activity.

7. There is no demonstrable improvement or increase in the level of performance of athletes or others from the consumption of protein in excess of the Recommended Dietary Allowance.

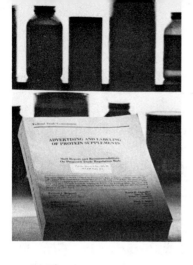

The Federal Trade Commission's report, *Advertising and Labeling of Protein Supplements,* points out that protein supplements are totally unnecessary for fitness-minded people. The study also notes that supplements usually cost more than an equivalent amount of protein-rich foods.

8. The consumption of protein, as such, has no benefit in weight reduction.

9. The "food energy" value of protein is derived from its caloric content alone. Protein itself does not remedy fatigue or lassitude. Once basic protein needs have been met, protein contributes to an individual's vigor, energy, alertness, strength, or endurance only to the extent of its caloric count.

10. The information currently required to be disclosed on protein supplements is not adequate for consumers.

Q. *If information from the government exists to show that protein supplements are unnecessary, why do fitness centers continue to sell them?*

A. The main reason many fitness centers sell protein supplements is to make money. These products can often be purchased in quantity by fitness centers for 50% or more below their retail selling price.

Of course, many managers of fitness centers, as well as a large number of the members, are believers in protein supplements. They sincerely think that athletic people need to consume protein powders and pills.

Once again, the use of protein supplements offers no significant nutritional benefits.

PROTEIN SUPPLEMENTS VS. PROTEIN-RICH FOODS

Q. *Are protein supplements better sources of protein than ordinary protein-rich foods?*

A. In order to answer this question, the following should be compared: protein content, protein quality, and cost per gram.

Current labeling practices often add to the difficulty facing the consumer who wishes to determine the protein content of a supplement. Supplement brand names will have within them a percentage or formula number that has no relationship to actual protein content of the product. For example, *Naturlabs Protein 95%* is 70% protein; *Pro-Glan 100* is 90% protein; *Super-Hi-Protein Formula 90 Tablets* are 82.7 or 83.7% protein; *Dr. Donbach's Formula 80* is 70% protein; and *Formula 94 Hi Protein* is 84% protein, according to information published in the Federal Trade Commission's January 15, 1979, staff report on *Advertising and Labeling of Protein Supplements*.

In addition to this labeling confusion, some explicit claims of protein content are "patently inaccurate," according to the same FTC document. Chemical analyses to determine the protein content of a number of supplements were conducted by the U.S. Department of Agriculture's Western Regional Research Laboratory. "The results of these tests showed that the majority of protein supplements analyzed claimed a greater protein content in labeling and advertising than the product, in the form sold, actually contained," states the report. "For example, the label for Radiance Products 'Glan-Pro Tablets' states that the product is 90 percent protein whereas analysis found the product to be 58.4 percent in the form sold and 62.1 percent on a dry basis. . . . Similarly, an advertisement for Shaklee's 'Instant Protein' claims that the product is 96 percent protein (dry basis) whereas analysis found the product to be 58 percent protein in the form sold and 59.8 percent protein on a dry basis. . . ."

"An even greater complex of claims is presented in determining the protein content of Superior Health Vitamins and Health Food's 'Super Pro-Gest,'" the report continues. "The front label of this supplement states the product is 'prepared from 100 percent Collagen protein.' The label's

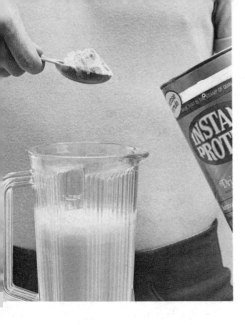

Protein drinks are popular among many athletes. But contrary to this practice, athletes do not need to supplement their diets with protein. Furthermore, the labels on many supplements are filled with discrepancies.

ingredient panel states the product contains '15 grams of protein hydrolysate from 90 percent animal protein.' Chemical analysis determined that the product contains 37.1 percent protein in the form sold. . . ."

Since protein supplements are explicitly promoted as concentrated sources of protein, the cost of these products is important to the consumer. Many buyers are under the impression that protein supplements are a less expensive form of protein than are meat, eggs, or other protein-rich foods.

Advertisements of some supplements promote their products as economical sources of protein. They will call a product, for example, a "best protein buy." Or they will claim that the purchaser has "nothing to lose but the high cost" of the food alternate.

As the chart on page 72 demonstrates, the cost per gram of usable protein (a measure of quality as well as quantity of protein) provided by protein supplements is generally much higher than the cost of protein provided by ordinary foods.

Protein supplements are more costly per ounce than protein-rich foods. The supplements are, in general, made of a lower-quality protein.

In the final analysis, protein supplements are *not* better sources of protein than ordinary protein-rich foods.

Cost Comparison Usable Protein From Ordinary Foods and Usable Protein From Protein Supplements

Ordinary Protein-Rich Foods	Cost Per Ten Grams Usable Protein	Protein Supplements	Cost Per Ten Grams Usable Protein
Non-fat powdered skimmed milk	7.1¢	Thompson 90% Protein Powder	15.1¢
Eggs, large	10.6¢	Schiff Hi-Protamine	18.4¢
Milk, whole fluid	14.0¢	Dr. Donbach's GL-Pro	24.4¢
Hamburger	14.9¢	Kalamino Amino Acid	25.6¢
Beef liver	15.7¢	H&J Formula 94 Hi Protein	25.8¢
Chicken	16.2¢	Hoffman's Superior Hi-Protein Tablets	27.8¢
Tuna	16.9¢	Nature's Plus Pre-Pro 15 Liquid	35.7¢
Peanut butter	18.6¢	NF Factors Protesoy	37.6¢
Cheddar cheese	20.0¢	Rich Life Hydrolized Protein Supplement	52.9¢
Sirloin beefsteak	32.7¢	American Dietary Labs Pro Gram Tablets	53.1¢
		Shaklee Instant Protein Powder	57.0¢
		Neo-Life Super Ease Hi Protein	62.4¢
		Malabar 100% Organ Meat	71.4¢
		LPP Predigested Protein with Vitamin C	102.6¢
		Unipro Development Unipro 9	362.8¢

Computation of costs of usable protein from ordinary foods were based on USDA Food and Protein Cost Tables for April 1975. Protein supplement costs were taken from 1975 product labels.

PROTEIN DANGERS

Q. *What are the risks of taking large amounts of protein?*

A. There is substantial danger in giving infants concentrated protein supplements. A protein feeding representing 20–40% of the calories ingested will put an infant at risk of becoming dehydrated.

Danger exists for persons with liver or kidney disorders. The amount of protein that may put a patient at risk varies inversely with the degree of liver or kidney malfunction.

Studies conducted on animals also suggest that excessive amounts of dietary protein may be damaging to the liver and kidneys of athletes. The metabolism and excretion of these nonstorable protein loads imposes serious stress and may cause excessive growth of these very important organs.

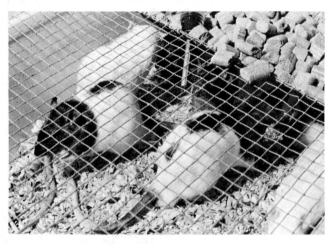

Laboratory rats that are fed high-protein diets for extended periods of time have shorter life spans than rats fed balanced diets. Much of the reduced life span is related to the additional stress a high-protein diet has on a rat's liver and kidneys.

Many obese people became aware of the dangers of liquid protein supplements several years ago. Government investigators suspect that at least 58 reported deaths may be linked to the diet that combines fasting with the use of liquid protein. Most of the liquid protein diets sold over the counter are not properly fortified with minerals, particularly potassium. A deficiency of potassium can lead to sudden death. The liquid protein diet may also produce great shifts in body water and electrolytes, causing cardiac arrest.

PSYCHOLOGICAL BENEFITS

Q. *What about the athlete who has been taking protein pills for the last two months and notes an improved performance? How can this be explained?*

A. Many factors could be responsible for improved performance. Chances are that the athlete's success was a result of improved skill, condition, strength, or the natural maturation process, and not protein pills. If the protein pills did anything at all, it was psychological. When an athlete who is approaching maximum performance in his specialty *believes* that he has a secret weapon (protein pills), he might be motivated to exert extra effort and discipline to better his performance. Self-confidence derived from consuming a supplement alleged to have remarkable powers could make a difference in championship competition. But if this is the only contribution that large amounts of protein pills are making, then such a nutritional program cannot be justified considering its cost and possible health hazard.

Prior to the liquid protein boom in 1976, many bodybuilders and weight lifters had been consuming the liquid protein supplements for years. Fortunately, they were also eating other foods. Scientists who have analyzed the dark syrup liquids say they contain low-quality, partly digested protein derived from cattle hides and tendons. Artificial flavor and saccharin are added to disguise the otherwise horrid taste.

PROTEIN AND ENERGY

Q. *The terms* power-packed *protein and* go-power *protein are frequently used in advertising food products. Isn't this misleading?*

A. Yes, this type of advertising is misleading. This is one of the things, in fact, that the Federal Trade Commission is trying to regulate.

Although proteins can be used as energy sources when necessary, carbohydrates and fats are better energy sources because they are more easily utilized in the body and less expensive than protein foods. The promotion of power-packed or go-power protein, therefore, is a sales gimmick.

ALL-MEAT DIET

Q. *Some athletes advocate a diet of meat and vitamin-mineral supplement. Is this healthy?*

A. Although it is possible to exist on a diet of meat and a vitamin-mineral supplement for a period of time, it is surely not recommended. The almost complete abstinence from eating carbohydrates imposes a number of serious hardships on the body:

1. The body requires a small amount of carbohydrates for use as a source of energy for the brain and nervous tissue.

2. A disturbance in the acid-base balance and a tendency toward acidosis also would occur. The estimated daily need for about 125 grams of carbohydrate would have to be synthesized from fat and from amino acid breakdown.

3. The almost complete absence of roughage would interfere with digestion, absorption, and excretion.

4. This type of diet would also be dangerous to anyone susceptible to gout or to uric acid kidney stones, as well as anyone having elevated blood fats and cholesterol.

PROTEIN AND BODYBUILDING

Q. *Since bodybuilders and weight lifters are interested in developing muscular size and strength, they should consume extra protein. Right?*

A. It might seem that extra protein would be needed for building large muscles, especially since muscles supposedly are made of protein. But only 22% of muscle is actually protein.

What does this mean to a weight lifter or bodybuilder? Simply that it takes very little protein to produce a pound of muscle, particularly since so little muscular growth actually takes place within a given 24-hour period. A normal diet will supply a bodybuilder or weight lifter with more than enough protein to build muscles.

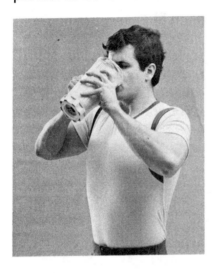

Bodybuilders and weight lifters should not be misled by food supplement advertising that says, "you need to add protein supplements to your diet for larger muscles." A normal diet supplies more than enough protein to build larger muscles—given that the muscles first are stimulated to grow through proper exercise.

PROTEIN AND SPECIAL VIRTUES

Q. *Some athletes eat large quantities of certain protein foods such as milk, meat, or eggs. Do any of these protein foods offer special virtues to them?*

A. No single food provides all essential nutrients. Any diet that contains large amounts of a single food will tend to be unbalanced or deficient in one or more nutrients. The best diet will always include a wide variety of foods.

RAW-EGG CONSUMPTION

Q. *Some people like to mix several raw eggs into a milk shake. Is this recommended?*

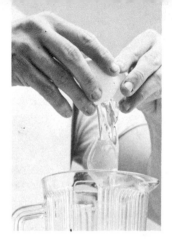

An egg is an excellent source of protein, vitamin A, and iron, and a good source of riboflavin and vitamin D. From both a nutritional and safety point of view, an egg should be eaten cooked rather than raw.

A. Although the addition of raw eggs can improve the flavor and nutritional value of a milk shake, this should be avoided because of the possibility of illness from contaminated eggs. Salmonella organisms, which cause food poisoning, can *remain* on the outside of the eggs even after washing. Invisible cracks in the shell may permit passage of the disease organism into the egg. Nutritionally, raw eggs are less desirable because they contain avidin (neutralized in cooking), which destroys biotin, a B vitamin. The usual methods of cooking eggs assure a safe product. An individual who wants to add an egg to a milk shake should soft-boil it first.

LIVER AS A FOOD

Q. *It has been said that liver is a high-protein food. How often should it be eaten?*

A. Liver is one of the best all-around foods for fitness-minded people. It is an excellent source of protein, vitamin A, the B vitamins, and iron. For this reason, nutritionists have advised people to eat liver frequently or about once every two weeks.

Many people, however, do not like the flavor of liver. If an individual is in this group, he also can select a nutritious diet from other foods. For example: (1) poultry, fish, meat, eggs, milk, and milk products provide high-quality protein; (2) meats, egg yolks, dried fruits, green leafy vegetables, and enriched and whole-grain cereals provide iron; (3) meats, milk, and cereals contain B vitamins; (4) deep yellow and green vegetables, whole milk, butter, and margarine provide

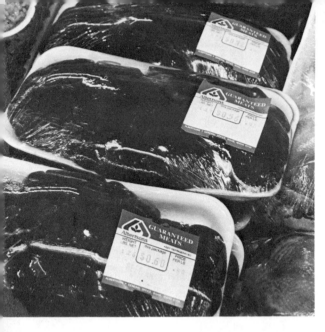

Liver is a highly nutritious food that all athletes should learn to enjoy.

vitamin A. If a person enjoys liver and eats it frequently, the assurance of adequate nutrition may be somewhat more certain but not necessarily more adequate than for a person who makes proper selections from other nutritious foods available to him.

VEGETARIANS AND PROTEIN

Q. How much does a vegetarian really have to worry about protein?

A. A lot depends on the specifics of the vegetarian's beliefs. Foods that are acceptable differ among vegetarians:

1. A pure, or strict, vegetarian diet excludes all foods of animal origin—meat, poultry, fish, eggs, and dairy products.

2. A lacto-vegetarian diet includes dairy products but excludes meat, poultry, fish, and eggs.

3. An ovo-lacto-vegetarian diet includes eggs and dairy products but excludes meat, poultry, and fish.

These distinctions are important because the complexity of selecting a nutritionally adequate vegetarian diet depends on the restrictiveness of the diet. For instance, the strict vegetarian must be careful to select foods that provide the nutrients

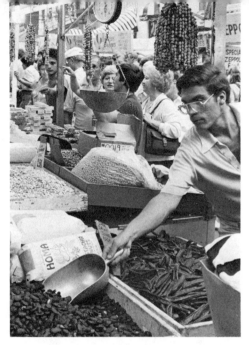

To obtain adequate protein on a daily basis, a vegetarian should consume multiple servings of grains, legumes, nuts, and seeds.

supplied by eggs and dairy products as well as meat. The ovo-lacto-vegetarian need be concerned only about including sources of nutrients commonly found in meat.

A daily guide for a meatless diet centers around sensible selections from four food groups: (1) grains, legumes, nuts, and seeds; (2) vegetables; (3) fruit; and (4) milk and eggs. Six servings a day from the first group (grains, legumes, nuts, and seeds) will provide most of the protein a person needs.

5

fats

FATS DEFINED

Q. *What are fats?*

A. Fats are a class of nutrients called lipids. The physical properties that distinguish most lipids from other compounds are their oiliness and their inability to dissolve in water. The lipid group includes fats, fatty acids, phospholipids, waxes, and nonphosphorylated lipids.

Most dietary lipids are fats or fatty acids. Phospholipids are a minor component of meat, and waxes are rare in foods. Although nonphosphorylated lipids account for little of the total diet, this group includes important *sterols,* such as *cholesterol* and vitamin D. Many of the male and female sex hormones are nonphosphorylated lipids.

Q. *What are fats made of?*

A. The main components of fats in food and in the body are fatty acids. Butter, for example, contains more than 29

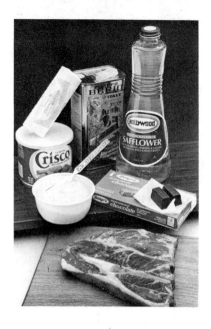

Fats are a part of every meal. Some fatty foods are familiar to everyone: margarine, butter, lard, vegetable oils, and beef fat. Unsweetened chocolate is also a fat-rich food—more than 50% of its calories are from fat.

fatty acids. The difference in taste of fats depends on which fatty acids predominate. The distribution of fatty acids also dictates the temperature at which a fat melts. This determines whether fats are solid or liquid at room temperature. Regardless of the fatty acid composition, all fats and oils contain nine calories per gram.

Fat is the most concentrated form of calories. One small pat of butter added to the portion of bread above, increases the calories of this snack threefold.

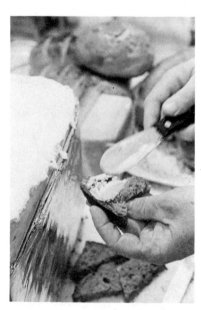

SOURCES OF FAT

Q. *What are the primary sources of fat in the average American's diet?*

A. The chief sources are milk, butter, cheese, margarine, meat, fish, and cooking oils. Most people are conscious of ingesting fat when they eat butter or margarine or the visible fat with meat; however, they are not conscious of "invisible" fat. Lean beef contains about 8% or more of invisible fat. In fact, choice grades of meat contain more fat or marbling than poorer grades. Foods such as vegetable oils and lard are 100% fat, while most fruits and vegetables contain less than 1% fat. The listing below shows the fat content of some common foods.

Average Fat Content of Typical Foods*

1.	Oils, shortenings	100%
2.	Butter, margarine	80%
3.	Most nuts	60%
4.	Peanut butter, bacon, donuts	50%
5.	Cheese, beef roasts	33%
6.	Lunch meat, franks	27%
7.	Lean pork, ice cream, cakes, pies	13%
8.	Most fish, lean lamb	7%
9.	Milk, shellfish, plain rolls	3%
10.	Most breads	1%

* Shown as a percentage of total weight

Oil is a common name for a food fat that is liquid at room temperature.

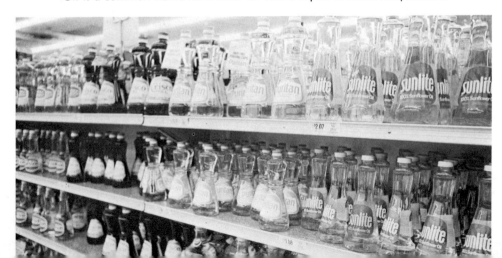

IMPORTANCE OF FAT

Q. *Is fat essential to a balanced diet?*

A. Yes. Fats are necessary to the life of all cells. At least one fatty acid, linoleic acid, is a dietary essential. Linoleic acid cannot be made by the human body, although all other fatty acids can be made in the body from this one. Thus, a dietary source of linoleic acid is essential for life. In its absence, a fatty acid deficiency develops, resulting first in minor symptoms such as scaly skin and sore spots.

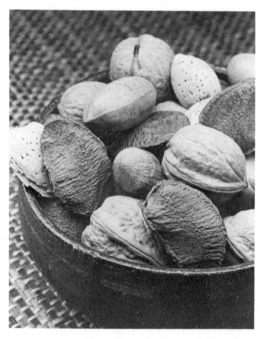

A dietary source of linoleic acid is essential for life. Salad and cooking oils, margarine, and nuts—especially walnuts— are a rich source of linoleic acid.

Excellent sources of linoleic acid are black walnuts, avocados, and vegetable oils such as safflower, corn, and soybean. Meats, such as bacon, ham, pork, and beef, are fair sources.

Q. *Other than the importance of linoleic acid, are there additional reasons why fat is essential in the diet?*

A. Fats and fat-containing foods are of value in the diet for several other reasons:

- As carriers of fat-soluble vitamins A, D, E, and K, and as an aid to their absorption in the intestine.
- As a concentrated source of energy and as a builder of fat stores in the body.
- For satiety value.
- For making foods appetizing and flavorful.
- For providing various functional properties to cooked and processed foods.

DEFINITIONS

Q. *Much confusion exists about cholesterol and such adjectives as* saturated, unsaturated, polyunsaturated, hydrogenated, *and* partially hydrogenated *when applied to salad oils, cooking oils, margarines, and shortening. What do they all mean?*

A. *Cholesterol* is a fat that animal cells (including man) can synthesize from building blocks provided by the breakdown of dietary carbohydrates and fats. It is made and used by most cells in the body and is required for optimal health. Cholesterol is not found in plants.

Saturated fats have all bonds in their carbon chains filled or saturated with hydrogen and are usually solids at room temperature. Animal fats are primarily saturated. Consumption of too much of these saturated fats over a period of years is believed to be a possible cause of cardiovascular or heart disease.

Unsaturated fats have bonds on their carbon chains that are not filled or are unsaturated with hydrogen. These places of unsaturation form double bonds between carbon atoms in their chain. Unsaturated fats are usually liquids called oils at room temperature and are generally derived from vegetable sources such as peanuts, cottonseeds, and soybeans.

Polyunsaturated fats are unsaturated fats having two or more places in the carbon chains that are not filled with hydrogen. These polyunsaturated fats are required by man, but man cannot make them. They must be present in the diet.

Hydrogenated fats or oils are fats that have been subjected to hydrogenation — a process whereby hydrogen is added to the fat, filling its unsaturated bonds. Such a process is said to produce a hardened fat because it typically converts an oil partially or completely to a fat or a solid. Fats that are solids at room temperature are called *fats* whereas fats that are liquids at room temperature are called *oils*.

Partially hydrogenated fats have had a portion or part of their unsaturated bonds filled with hydrogen. Since hydrogenation is a gradual process filling more and more unsaturated bonds with hydrogen, it can be stopped at any point so that the oil's hardness (or melting point) can be made to order.

Due to the high cost or inaccessibility of butter during World War II, hardened vegetable oils or margarines began to be used as spreads. Although the hydrogenation process converts an expensive oil to a marketable margarine, it also destroys, at least partially, its nutritional value, by converting the essential polyunsaturated fat to a *nonessential* saturated fat. Since the proportion of these two fats is critical to a fat's nutritional value, one day the process of hydrogenation will be regulated or controlled in such a way as to make the most nutritious yet marketable margarine. Another way of improving a fat's nutritional value is to shorten the chain length or select oils that have the desirable chain length.

The majority of the edible oils in this country are obtained from corn, cottonseed, soybeans, olives, and peanuts. They are used in a wide variety of food products ranging from cooking oils to margarines. Several margarine manufacturers have prepared products for partial hydrogenation that are supposed to have all the characteristics of margarine yet contain significant quantities of unaltered vegetable oils.

OVERCONSUMPTION OF FAT

Q. *Are Americans eating about the right amount of fat, too much, or too little?*

A. Since 1900 the percentage of calories represented by fat in the diet has increased from 30% to well over 40%. In certain groups, such as male college students and businessmen, it exceeds 50%. At one time it was thought that the replacement of starches by fats, calorie for calorie, was a matter of no consequence. Shortly after World War II, however, the work of Dr. Ancel Keys suggested that a high fat intake might be associated with a greater prevalence of heart disease. Over the past 25 years, evidence has accumulated indicating that elevated levels of cholesterol in the blood—from large amounts of saturated fat in the diet—were accompanied by an increase in cardiovascular disease.

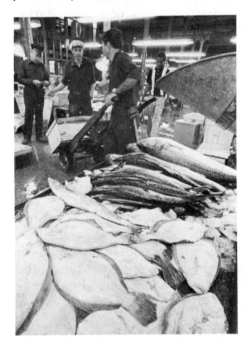

Fish generally has less fat and cholesterol than meat and consequently fewer calories. It is also rich in some minerals.

In contrast, it appears that polyunsaturated fats decrease the level of blood cholesterol. There is some evidence that proper exercise seems to decrease blood cholesterol. Uncorrected high blood pressure, overweight, the presence or absence of certain trace minerals, stress, lack of sleep, cigarette smoking, and diabetes may promote heart attacks and strokes. It is suggested that persons at risk for any reason reduce their fat intake, if high, to no more than 30% of the total calories.

FACTS ABOUT CHOLESTEROL

Q. *Recently the Food and Nutrition Board suggested that the dangers of dietary cholesterol may have been overstated. What is the truth about cholesterol?*

A. Some of the risk factors pertaining to cholesterol are still controversial. Almost all researchers, however, agree that cholesterol is somehow associated with heart disease, though quite likely not an essential condition or cause of it. As Dr. William B. Kannel says, "Cholesterol seems to be the thread running through the web of circumstances that results in a heart attack or stroke." The famous Framingham Heart Study indicates that a man with a total cholesterol of 260 (mg. per 100 ml.) has a risk for a heart attack three times that of a man whose count is under 195. The risk becomes five-fold at a cholesterol count of 310.

The correlation between total cholesterol level and the risk for heart disease has been muddied by the knowledge that not all the cholesterol reflected in the total count is bad. The form of cholesterol known as HDL (high-density lipoprotein) is associated with a *decreased* risk for heart disease. More information is now being gathered on good versus bad cholesterol.

Evidence also shows that low-fat diets do not *always* improve the cholesterol pattern. Again, almost all experts would agree that dietary changes would be good for some people. This is especially true for those with a strong family history of premature heart disease, those with known heart disease, and those who are obese. While these groups encompass many Americans, it must be admitted that there are other Americans who do not need to restrict dietary fats and cholesterol.

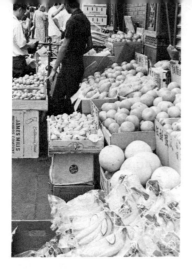

One way for Americans to lower their dietary cholesterol is to consume more fruits and vegetables. Fruits and vegetables are virtually cholesterol-free.

After all the evidence is considered, the prudent recommendation is that most Americans should lower the amounts of fat and cholesterol in their diets. This is still the best advice to follow.

NONDAIRY CREAMERS

Q. *Is it better for a person to consume nondairy creamers than cream in beverages?*

A. Nondairy creamers usually are made from plant oils. They do not contain cholesterol, as does cream. The plant oil most commonly used is coconut. This is a saturated fat. If the reduction of saturated fats in the diet is the goal, nonfat dry or liquid skimmed milk would be a better substitute for cream. The nondairy creamers contain about 11 calories per teaspoon. Cream contains about 14 calories per teaspoon.

VEGETABLE OILS

Q. *What is the difference between the untreated vegetable oils sold in health food stores and regular vegetable oils?*

A. These untreated oils are cold-pressed from such plants as safflower, corn, cotton, and soybean. They are bottled without preservatives or additives. Taken in the proper amounts, these oils can provide a valuable source of polyunsaturated fatty acids in the diet. The nutritional value of the vegetable oils, however, is easily destroyed when left to stand

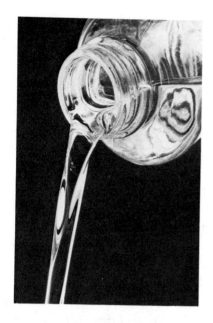

Vegetable oils, which are used in cooking and preparing salad dressings, provide a valuable source of polyunsaturated fatty acids.

or when heated. Untreated oils should be purchased in small quantities and not heated for they are extremely perishable. Furthermore, the Department of Agriculture has been unable to find any harmful effects that are produced from using the common vegetable oils that do contain preservatives.

"FATTENING" FOODS

Q. *What about the consumption of "fattening" foods such as potatoes, gravy, and candies? Should they be limited in the diet?*

A. It is a misnomer to label any food as "fattening." The total caloric intake each day makes the difference, not the presence of one particular food. If a person ate three cups of mashed potatoes (about 735 calories) every day and excluded all other foods, he would lose weight. Why? Because the total number of calories consumed would be less than the calories expended. There are foods that only supply energy and no other nutrients. These foods should be limited if a person is having trouble losing weight and still meeting all his nutrient requirements.

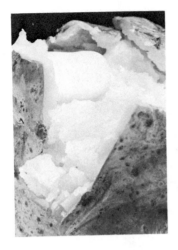

A large baked potato contains fair amounts of niacin, thiamine, vitamin B_6, vitamin C, and protein—and only 140 calories. But add one tablespoon of butter to that low-calorie potato and the calories jump to 240.

FAT AND MUSCLE

Q. *What is the difference between fat and muscle?*

A. If we chemically analyzed a pound of fat and a pound of muscle, we would discover some interesting facts. Both fat and muscle contain water, lipids (fats), and protein, in varying amounts as follows:

	Calories	Water	Lipids	Protein
Muscle	600	70%	7%	22%
Fat	3,500	22%	72%	6%

An individual should not forget that a pound of fat has 3,500 calories while a pound of muscle contains only 600 calories. Most of muscle is water, whereas fatty tissue is mainly composed of fat.

FATS BEFORE SPORTS

Q. *Should the athlete restrict his consumption of fats, fried foods, and oily dressings?*

A. The human body needs a certain amount of fat for proper functioning. Fats in the diet are carriers of the fat-soluble vitamins A, D, E, and K, and one fatty acid, linoleic.

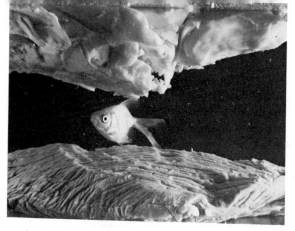

Muscle is much denser than fat as this photograph dramatically shows. A pound of muscle sinks to the bottom of an aquarium, while an equal amount of fat floats.

These are essential nutrients. Furthermore, fat provides flavor, satisfaction, variety, and a concentrated form of energy. When fats enter the intestinal tract, they cause the release of a hormone, enterogastrone, which slows down the emptying time of the stomach. Although this provides a longer period of satiety after a meal, there are times when slow stomach emptying may be undesirable and fat intake should be limited. A pregame meal is such a situation.

Most fats are digested at about the same rate whether they are in the form of butter, margarine, salad dressings, shortening, or in the natural fat content of food. The normal athlete can successfully digest food fried in fat that has not been burned or that does not contain other contaminants. Moderate amounts of fried foods are not taboo for the athlete.

A close-up of a beef chuck steak shows the intermingling of fat with muscle. Most of the calories from this meat come from fat rather than protein. A broiled six-ounce chuck steak provides 490 calories—290 from fat and 200 from protein.

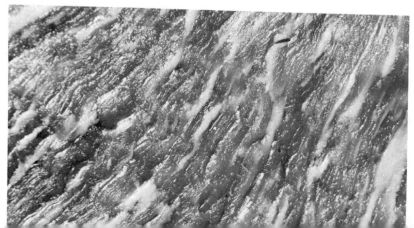

ACNE

Q. *Should a person with acne avoid certain foods such as chocolate, nuts, and milk?*

A. No. Acne is not caused by improper diet. Chocolate does not cause acne. Peanuts do not cause acne. Oil-rich foods do not cause acne. Milk does not cause acne. According to the American Medical Association's Committee on Cutaneous Health and Cosmetics, acne is caused primarily by hyperactive oil glands in the skin. The oil glands oversecrete and become plugged, thus producing acne. The hyperactivity of these glands is presumably caused by hormonal imbalance during adolescence, especially in the early processes of maturation.

For treating acne, the American Medical Association has recommended frequent and thorough, but not abrasive, cleaning of the skin with a good-quality soap and hot water. Medications used under the direction of a physician also can be useful.

Although diet alone will neither clear the skin nor prevent acne, a well-balanced diet is important to skin health. Since nutrient demands are greatest during the growth phase of adolescence, every effort must be made to assure a good supply of calories, proteins, vitamins, and minerals. To deviate from a balanced diet in an attempt to clear up acne is not only foolish; it is very hazardous.

6

carbohydrates

DIFFERENCE BETWEEN PROTEINS, FATS, AND CARBOHYDRATES

Q. *What is the difference between proteins, fats, and carbohydrates?*

A. There are essentially three kinds of foods that the body uses for fuel or maintenance (building and replacing cells):

1. *Proteins,* from meat, poultry, fish, dairy products, eggs, nuts, and some grains.

2. *Fats,* from meat, oils, nuts and grains, and milk products.

3. *Carbohydrates,* the starches and sugars in fruits and vegetables and in bread, pastries, and everything else made with flour and/or sugar.

These three types of foods, while being distinct, are still chemical cousins. All three have a chemical spine that is composed of carbon atoms, with arms of hydrogen and oxygen. But proteins are far more complex than carbohydrates

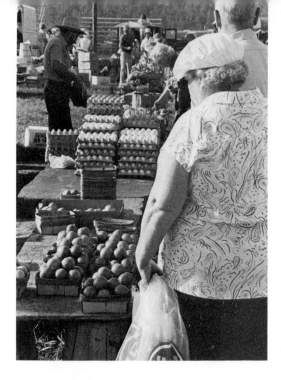

In the minds of many people there are two magical pathways for food in the body. Carbohydrates go straight into the fat, and proteins go to the muscles. These are fallacies.

and fats. Proteins also contain nitrogen and sometimes sulfur. Fats have far less oxygen and thus contain more calories than proteins and carbohydrates. Carbohydrates are the easiest to digest.

CARBOHYDRATES DEFINED

Q. *What are carbohydrates?*
A. Carbohydrates are made up of carbon, hydrogen, and oxygen. They are assembled in green plants by the light from the sun working on carbon dioxide and water. Carbohydrates are found in our food supply as starches, sugars, and fiber.

OCCURRENCE OF CARBOHYDRATES

Q. *How widespread are carbohydrates in foods?*
A. In nature carbohydrates are more plentiful than all other organic materials combined. This is because all plants are composed primarily of carbohydrates. The plant's supporting structure, cellulose, and its storage form of energy, starch, are carbohydrates.

Plants are able to synthesize carbohydrates, fats, proteins, and vitamins from water, soil minerals, and carbon dioxide using the energy from the sun in the process called photosynthesis. Most of the nutrients required by man must be obtained in the diet either from plants or from other animals that have consumed plants.

We can therefore speak of energy conversion rates and efficiencies. Plants convert energy much more efficiently per acre than animals. Thus, plant foods are less expensive. Although the carbohydrates, fats, minerals, and vitamins are of high quality, the protein synthesized by plants is not ideally suited for man and is considered to be of poor quality.

Cellulose, which is the plant's supporting structure, is the grazing animal's most important dietary carbohydrate. Man is not able to digest cellulose and is unable to derive energy from this carbohydrate. Starch, which is the plant's storage form of energy, is man's most common form of dietary carbohydrate. It supplies more than half of the energy sources in the American diet.

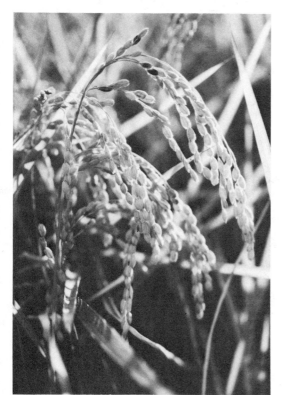

Rice grows in moist tropical climates. Because of its importance in the diet of the populous countries of the East, rice is consumed more than any other grain in the world. (Photo by David Cecil)

Common dietary carbohydrates are starch from plants; table sugar or sucrose, which is refined, or pure sugar prepared from sugar cane or sugar beets; milk sugar or lactose, which is synthesized in the mammary gland; malt sugar or maltose prepared from various plants; glucose or dextrose, which is found in many fruits; and cellulose. Glucose is the carbohydrate that circulates in the blood and enters cells as one of its energy sources. Although cellulose or fiber does not provide energy for man, it is a useful dietary constituent because it supplies most of the bulk of the diet. Bulk aids in intestinal function and regularity of bowel movements.

Glycogen is man's storage form of carbohydrate and is found in muscle and liver. When these storage sites are filled, any additional amounts of carbohydrate consumed in the diet are converted to fat and stored as such. The body can store an almost unlimited amount of energy as fat—100 times more energy in the form of fat than it can in the form of carbohydrate (glycogen).

Average Carbohydrate Content of Typical Foods*

1. Sugar, honey	99%
2. Most dry cereals	80%
3. Cookies, crackers	73%
4. Dried fruits, jams	70%
5. Bread	50%
6. Grains, noodles, potatoes	25%
7. Legumes, beans, peas	18%
8. Fresh fruits	12%
9. Leafy vegetables	4%

* Shown as a percentage of total weight

FUNCTIONS OF CARBOHYDRATES

Q. *How do carbohydrates function in the human body?*

A. The main function of dietary carbohydrates in the body is the provision of energy. Since other nutrients can also provide energy, health may be maintained with diets that differ greatly in their carbohydrate content. Some people survive with diets made up almost entirely of protein and fats, while other people live with diets that are over 80% carbohydrate. Carbohydrate intake is influenced primarily by economic factors. Lower-income families tend to consume more carbohydrates, and higher-income families consume more proteins and fats. On the average, carbohydrate consumption has decreased in the United States since 1900.

While life can be maintained with little carbohydrate material in the diet, there is considerable evidence that a liberal intake of carbohydrate is advisable. Presumably, this is due more to the dangers or toxicity of high-fat diets and less to the special merits of dietary carbohydrates. An energy source is obviously required in the diet and there are three choices: carbohydrates, fats, or proteins. Carbohydrates present in various fruits are the preferred sources of energy by the body since they are easily absorbed and require less alteration prior to the release of their energy. If the dietary source of energy is one other than protein, then the expensive proteins can be used more appropriately as building blocks and will not have to be burned to supply energy.

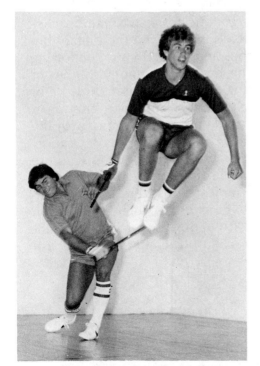

The preferred fuel for participation in racquetball and other movement-related sports is carbohydrates. (Photo by Inge Cook)

Since too many saturated fats in the diet have been shown to be linked to cardiovascular disease, they must be kept at a reasonable level. But saturated fats are a useful and desirable component in the diet if they are consumed in moderation and balanced with the amount of polyunsaturated fats in the diet.

So a mix of approximately two to one of carbohydrates to fats, with an emphasis on the polyunsaturated fats, seems to be the desirable energy source. Protein is a very important dietary constituent, but it will not be used as efficiently as it should be without a nonprotein energy source in the diet.

In summary, the main contributions of carbohydrate-rich foods are to:

- Provide an economical energy supply;
- Furnish some proteins, minerals, and vitamins (whole grains, legumes, and potatoes);
- Add flavor (sugar) to foods and beverages.

QUICK-ENERGY FOODS

Q. *What are the best quick energy foods for the athlete?*

A. A study reported by Dr. Dale O. Nelson of Utah State University in *Scholastic Coach* indicates how some coaches responded to this question. Nelson surveyed the dietary beliefs of various athletic coaches and noted that the following foods were thought to be the best quick energy sources or precontest meals for competing athletes: oranges, dextrose or glucose, honey, vitamin C tablets, chocolate, Coke, and sugar. These foods are composed mainly of carbohydrates, with the exception of vitamin C and chocolate, and are good energy sources. Although some of the coaches and athletes who use these products claim they provide almost immediate surges of energy, research in this area indicates that only athletes who compete in long endurance-type contests, such as marathon running and skiing, benefit from the use of certain high-carbohydrate diets. Dr. Peter V. Karpovich, prominent physiologist at Springfield College, and Dr. P. Astrand of Sweden believe than most sports are of such short duration that there is no apparent physiological benefit from precontest meals. The energy used in competition ordinarily comes from food consumed from several days to two weeks prior to the game or contest.

PRECOMPETITION MEALS

Q. *Are there any special foods an athlete should eat prior to competition?*

A. No, there are no special foods. What an athlete eats on the day of competition has little to do with the production of energy for that day. It makes good sense, however, for the athlete to pay attention to certain guidelines:

1. Energy intakes should be adequate to ward off feelings of hunger or weakness during competition. Although the food eaten prior to competition has little to do with immediate energy expenditure, it can give the athlete a feeling of strength and security.

2. The necessity of urinary or bowel excretion during performance can be serious or even disabling. For this reason, meals that include large amounts of protein foods, bulky foods, or highly spiced foods should be avoided before competition or consumed in small quantities.

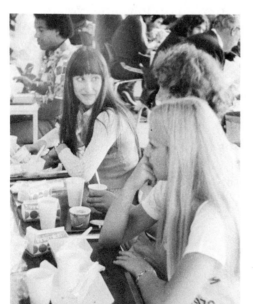

The precompetition meal for an athlete should take place at least three hours prior to the starting time. (Photo by Ellington Darden)

3. The meal should be eaten at least three hours prior to starting time to allow for digestion to take place.

4. Fluid intakes prior to, during, and after prolonged competition should guarantee an optimal state of hydration. This can be accomplished with various thirst drinks, fruit juices, and just plain water.

5. The precompetition meal should include food that the athlete is familiar with—food that he thinks will "make him win." All athletes should remember that eating can be as much psychological as it is physiological.

MOST EFFICIENT SOURCE OF ENERGY

Q. *Which nutrient does the body prefer for energy in athletic performance?*

A. The body prefers carbohydrates and fats as sources of energy over proteins. Early experiments suggested that the intensity of activity or work determined whether the body preferred fats or carbohydrates to satisfy its energy requirement. The body's preference for carbohydrates or fats as energy sources is about the same during mild exercise as at rest. As the athlete's activity increases to maximum, however, the more important the carbohydrate sources become, until finally all the energy is derived from carbohydrates. The preference for dietary carbohydrates depends on the intensity of activity and the oxygen supply to the working muscles: the more inadequate the oxygen supply, the greater the carbohydrate utilization.

Q. *How does the diet affect work metabolism for the athlete?*

A. This question has recently been investigated by a group of Swedish physiologists directed by Dr. Jonas Bergstrom. The amount of muscle glycogen in the quadriceps femoris muscle was monitored in men during heavy exercise and with various diets. Subjects were fed for three days on one of three diets, each providing 2,800 calories: (1) a typical mixed diet, (2) a

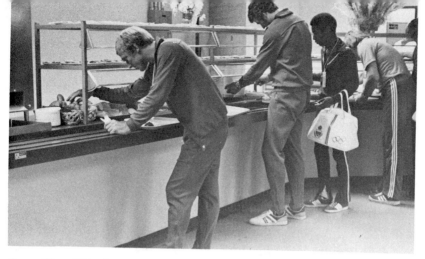

From 55 to 60% of an athlete's diet should be from carbohydrate-rich foods. (Photo by Ellington Darden)

diet containing protein and fats, and (3) a diet containing carbohydrates. After the subjects received one of the diets for three days, they were subjected to maximal work time with a work load demanding 75% of maximal aerobic power. Subjects consuming the carbohydrate diet were able to perform for 167 minutes. Those consuming the typical mixed diet tolerated the work load for 114 minutes. The subjects consuming the protein-fat diet tolerated the work load for 57 minutes.

A similar study was reported by this same research group working in St. Erik's Hospital, Stockholm, Sweden. Two subjects exercised on a bicycle ergometer, using only one leg, while the other leg was resting. After several hours of work, the glycogen content was analyzed in each leg, showing the exercised leg being emptied while the resting leg still had normal glycogen content. For the next three days the subjects consumed a diet composed mainly of carbohydrates. Although the glycogen content of the resting leg did not increase, the glycogen content of the exercising leg was more than twice as high as the rested leg. These workers concluded that different diets as well as activity have a marked influence on the capacity of muscles to recover from activity and to store energy.

This research suggests that *diet* as well as *activity* can markedly influence the metabolism of fats and carbohydrates.

On an adequate or balanced diet, the greater the exercise, the greater the relative energy yield from carbohydrates. Athletes should be aware that a high-carbohydrate diet improves the capacity for prolonged intensive exercise.

CARBOHYDRATE LOADING

Q. *Is carbohydrate loading prior to a marathon race beneficial to the runner?*

A. Carbohydrate loading does have a sound basis in theory and a reasonable body of experimental evidence to support it. It could supply a marathon runner with additional energy during the last portion of the race.

Q. *What is the proper way to carbohydrate load prior to a marathon race?*

A. Nutritional scientists recommend the following:

1. The individual should deplete his glycogen stores by exercising to exhaustion the same muscles that will be used in competition. This should be done about one week prior to the race.

2. For the next few days the diet should be almost exclusively fat and protein foods.

3. More exercise should be done three days prior to competition to ensure the absence of glycogen.

4. Then the athlete should add large quantities of carbohydrate to his diet for the next few days, or until the competition begins.

In the following table, the three phases show specific guidelines for a runner to follow prior to a Saturday morning marathon race.

Guidelines to Follow Prior to Marathon Race

Days Before Marathon	Training	Diet
Phase I { 8 days—Friday	normal	normal, mixed diet
7 days—Saturday	normal	normal, mixed diet
Phase II { 6 days—Sunday	long workout; 2½–3 hrs.	high protein and fat, low in carbohydrates
5 days—Monday	rest	high protein and fat, low in carbohydrates
4 days—Tuesday	light activity	high protein and fat, low in carbohydrates
3 days—Wednesday	hard one-hour workout to ensure no glycogen left	high carbohydrates, low in protein and fat
Phase III { 2 days—Thursday	rest	high carbohydrates, low in protein and fat
1 day—Friday	rest	high carbohydrates, low in protein and fat
Saturday	competition	high carbohydrates, low in protein and fat; weak sugar drinks during competition

The following foods are grouped under the headings of high-fat/protein and high-carbohydrate foods:

High-fat/protein foods: Meat, poultry, fish, cheese, eggs, nuts, butter. (It should be noted that aside from gelatin, which is almost pure protein, most protein foods contain high percentages of fat.)

High-carbohydrate foods: Sugar, honey, candy, bread, cereals, cookies, dried fruit, potatoes (not fried), fruit and fruit juices, jams and jellies, spaghetti, rice.

These nutritional guidelines apply only to the six days prior to competition. Diet and activity should be normal at all other times (Phase I). Phase II lasts for three days or 72 hours and is immediately followed by Phase III, which lasts for three days. Best results from the program will occur if the dietary recommendations are strictly practiced. And "strict" means 90% of the diet in Phase II should be fat/protein, and 90% of the diet in Phase III should be carbohydrate. It is also recommended that this six- or seven-day diet be practiced no more than *once every four months*. Complications could occur if it is practiced more frequently. Only a very important competition would merit such preparation.

The three-phase, carbohydrate-loading diet for marathon runners should be used only once every four months. (Photo by Art Gutierrez)

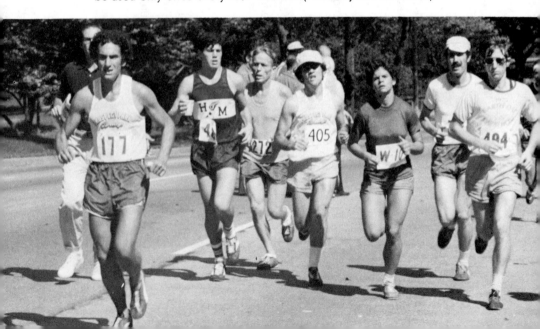

Q. *Does carbohydrate loading pose any risks?*

A. Some notes of warning have been sounded by physicians concerned over possible side effects of carbohydrate loading. They point out that water is deposited along with glycogen, which may cause the muscles to feel heavy and stiff.

Prostatitis, a swelling of the prostate gland accompanied by painful urination, is another potential complication. It is probably caused by inadequate fluid intake during carbohydrate loading. During the process, the athlete should drink more liquids than usual—at least eight 8-ounce glasses a day.

Severe carbohydrate restriction during the depletion phase of the loading process can cause ketosis, an accumulation of toxic substances in the blood that can lead to kidney damage. Ketosis also can be minimized by drinking at least eight glasses of fluid a day.

Older athletes with kidney and liver diseases are particularly susceptible to these side effects and should not attempt the depletion phase.

Even with its side effects, a carefully controlled program of carbohydrate loading can help the performance of marathon runners and other endurance athletes such as cyclers, skiers, rowers, and channel swimmers.

Q. *What about athletes such as tennis, racquetball, football, basketball, and baseball players? Will carbohydrate loading help them?*

A. Carbohydrate loading in noncontinuous sports or sports that involve a lot of stopping and starting has minimal effect on performance. Most athletes have enough glycogen stored in their livers and muscles (approximately 1,500 calories) for at least 60 minutes of vigorous continuous activity. The body's normal glycogen supply is more than enough for successful participation in tennis, racquetball, football, basketball, and baseball.

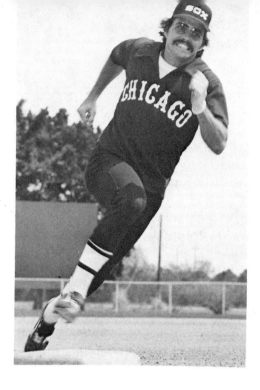

Baseball players are involved in noncontinuous activities during games. Rarely does a player run for more than five seconds. Carbohydrate loading prior to a baseball game is therefore unnecessary.

STARCHES AND CARBOHYDRATES

Q. *Are the terms starches and carbohydrates synonymous? Are starches digestible?*

A. These terms are not synonymous. Starches are carbohydrates, but not all carbohydrates are starches. *Carbohydrate* is a general term used to identify one of the basic classes of food components. Proteins, fats, vitamins, and minerals are other such general terms. Carbohydrates can be divided into two groups: (1) simple sugars, such as glucose or dextrose (monosaccharides) and common table sugar (disaccharides); and (2) complex carbohydrates, such as starch and cellulose (polysaccharides).

Starch is the storage form of sugar and is man's principal dietary carbohydrate. Fruits and their degree of sweetness **depend on the kind and amount of simple sugars produced when starch is broken down by ripening or cooking.**

In man, the energy from starch can be utilized only after it is broken down to simple sugar by digestive enzymes. The enzyme that is most important in the digestion of starch is amylase. It is secreted by the mouth and the pancreas, so starch digestion begins in the mouth, continues to a small extent in the stomach, and is completed in the small intestine. Since the digestive enzymes in saliva are thoroughly mixed with food by chewing, and since digestive enzymes can operate best on small particles of food, food should be well chewed before swallowing in order to provide for its maximum digestion and absorption.

ZERO-CARBOHYDRATE DIET

Q. *Would there be any value to a zero-carbohydrate diet?*

A. No! Carbohydrates contain four calories per gram. This is the same figure as proteins, which many people consider low in calories. Carbohydrates appear to be the near-exclusive food of the brain. Eating less than 400 calories of carbohydrates per day means that the individual must convert proteins into carbohydrates and this is not recommended by most nutritionists.

FIBER DEFINED

Q. *Recently, much has been written about the importance of dietary fiber. What exactly is fiber?*

A. Fiber can be defined as the cell walls of plant tissues. Crude fiber is what is left after a food sample has been treated by strong, hot acid and alkali. This is the only available laboratory technique for simulating physiological digestion. Dietary fiber is the term used for all the components of plants that are not broken down by enzymes in the digestive tract. Most foods contain more dietary fiber than crude fiber. For example, 100 grams of whole wheat bread contain 8.5 grams of dietary fiber, but only 1.5 grams of crude fiber. Food composition tables list crude fiber.

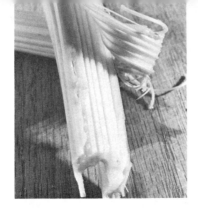

Raw vegetables, such as cauliflower, carrots, spinach, radishes, cabbage, and celery are high in fiber.

IMPORTANCE OF FIBER

Q. *Why is fiber important in nutrition?*

A. Scientists know that a high-fiber diet is helpful in preventing constipation. It also has been used successfully in treating diverticulosis, a condition in which abnormal pouches form in the walls of the large intestine.

Some people think that fiber may protect against a variety of diseases, including cancer, heart attacks, diabetes, gallstones, hemorrhoids, and obesity. Such claims rest on shaky ground, however.

Q. *How much fiber should a fitness-minded individual consume each day?*

A. There is no Recommended Dietary Allowance for fiber. Certain guidelines, however, should prove helpful.

Studies have found that the average American diet provides approximately four grams of crude fiber a day. Many nutritionists think that Americans would be wise to increase their consumption of crude fiber to at least six grams per day.

Many people should eat more high-fiber foods, such as fruits, vegetables, breads, and cereals. But the indiscriminate use of fiber, especially in purified form (bran), is not recommended. Wheat bran, for example, is high in phytate. Phytate has been shown to bind calcium, zinc, iron, and other trace elements, and thereby reduce their absorption into the blood.

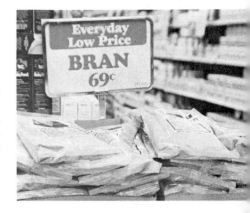

An individual will get enough fiber if he consumes a well-balanced diet that contains a variety of whole-grain breads and cereals as well as vegetables such as broccoli, carrots, peas, cabbage, salad greens and corn, and various fruits, especially apples, peaches, berries, pears, and bananas.

Approximate Crude Fiber Content Per Serving of Food

Food	Crude Fiber (grams/serving)
Cereal, ½–⅔ cup	
All-bran	3.0
40% bran	0.9
Wheat bran	0.8
Most other cooked or ready-to-eat cereals	0.3
Bread, 1 slice	
Whole wheat, pumpernickel	0.4
Raisin, rye, French, Italian, enriched white	0.05–0.2
Fruits, medium size or ½ cup	
Apple (with skin)	2.0
Watermelon	1.5
Prunes, dried peaches	1.5
Honeydew, bananas	1.0
Berries	1.0
Peaches, apricots, citrus fruits, fruit cocktail	0.5
Fruit juice	0.2
Vegetables, ½–⅔ cup	
Parsnips, peas, brussel sprouts	2.0
Pork'n beans	2.0
Beans, lima	1.5
Beans, kidney	1.0
Broccoli, carrots	1.0
Green beans, corn, celery, turnip, tomatoes, greens	0.5–1.0
Potato (with skin)	0.8
Potato chips, spinach	0.5
Nuts, ½ cup	1.0–2.0
Sunflower seeds, 1 cup	2.0

IRRITATING FOODS

Q. *Many coaches advise athletes to avoid irritating foods such as spices and bulky foods such as lettuce and bran. They in turn recommend bland and nonirritating foods. Is there any value to this advice?*

A. The ideas that coaches have about which foods are bland or irritating are usually based on unverified impressions, traditional lore, or their own particular experiences. Reliable studies on this subject fail to substantiate various popular beliefs concerning the effects of food on digestion. The discomfort or difficulties caused by various foods is largely an individual matter. Modification of eating habits should be based on the athlete's previous experiences.

While black pepper, chili pepper, cloves, and mustard seed may be irritating to some, there seems to be no reason for limiting the use of other spices such as paprika, cinnamon, allspice, mace, thyme, and sage. Lettuce, often considered a roughage or bulk-type vegetable, actually contains only 1.6–4.5% of indigestible fiber. Lettuce and other vegetables and fruits of even higher fiber content do not upset the process of digestion. On the contrary, fiber is necessary for normal intestinal function and regularity. These foods, however, do increase fecal bulk. They are best reduced in the 24 hours preceding the competition or athletic event.

ALCOHOL CONSUMPTION

Q. *What about the consumption of alcohol? Is it nutritious?*

A. Alcohol contains seven calories per gram. It is primarily a source of calories.

Alcohol is produced by the action of yeast on carbohydrates. The starting material may be fruit, palm or cactus juices, molasses or sugar, honey, milk, potatoes, or cereal grains. The flavor of the final product will vary accordingly, but the alcohol produced is the same: the simple compound, ethyl alchohol or ethanol. Because fermentation is a metabolic process, the process must be stopped before the resulting wine becomes vinegar.

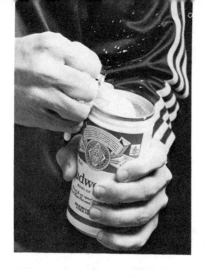

Beer is often said to contain valuable nutrients, such as B vitamins and protein. An adult male, however, would have to drink at least a six-pack of 12-ounce cans to meet his niacin requirements and nine six-packs to meet his protein requirements.

Hard liquors are produced by distillation, which concentrates the alchohol and separates it from the starting material. Thus, beer and wine contain some nutrients present in the original malted barley and fruit juice, but distilled spirits have no essential nutrients other than calories.

Q. *We have heard for years that alcohol should be avoided or consumed in moderation. Why is this so?*
A. Alcohol is metabolized in the liver, but the capacity is limited. Most individuals can metabolize about 50 calories of ethanol, or about a 12-ounce can of beer per one-and-a-half-hour time period. If alcohol is consumed at a rate faster than it can be metabolized, the level of alcohol builds up in body tissues and intoxication eventually results.
Alcohol can damage the liver. Chronic users have an increased risk of cirrhosis of the liver. In high concentration, alcohol is damaging to the lining of the intestinal tract and absorption of nutrients is affected adversely. Ultimately, overuse leads to degenerative changes in the brain and other parts of the nervous system.

Q. *Is it safe to drink alcoholic beverages?*
A. As long as alcoholic beverages are used in moderation and with awareness of the risks entailed, they can be consumed safely by most adults. Pregnant women, children, teenagers, and those on a noncompatible medication however, would be wise to avoid alcohol completely.

7

vitamins

VITAMINS DEFINED

Q. *What are vitamins?*

A. Vitamins are potent, indispensable, noncaloric compounds needed in very small amounts in the diet. They perform specific functions to promote growth and reproduction or to maintain health and life.

This definition separates the vitamins from proteins, fats, and carbohydrates. Unlike these nutrients, vitamins do not provide calories or energy. A fitness-minded individual may need several hundred grams of energy nutrients each day to maintain his body weight and support his activity. But vitamin needs are measured in thousandths (milligrams) or millionths (micrograms) of a gram.

DISCOVERY OF VITAMINS

Q. *How were vitamins discovered?*

A. Until the early 1900s it was thought that only carbohydrates, proteins, fats, minerals, and water were needed for

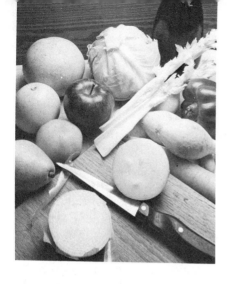

Fruits and vegetables are of value in the diet primarily as carriers of vitamins and minerals. A well-balanced diet should include at least four servings daily from the fruit and vegetable food group.

normal nutrition of humans and experimental animals. It had been known for centuries that liver, citrus fruits, and cod liver oil were able to prevent or cure specific human disorders. But most investigators paid little attention to some of the early hints of the existence of vitamins.

Credit for the discovery of vitamins cannot be given to any one person. Instead the honor goes to a few chemists and physiologists, working independently in several countries, who carefully studied why diets made of purified food ingredients were not able to support the life of experimental animals.

In 1905 a Dutch scientist, C. A. Pekelharing, fed small amounts of whey from milk to mice and concluded that milk had an unknown essential substance. He was certain that this substance not only occurred in milk but in all sorts of foodstuffs.

In England, at about the same time, F. G. Hopkins found that rats sickened and died on diets of pure protein, fat, carbohydrates, and minerals. Less than one-third of a teaspoon of milk per day added to this highly purified diet made all the difference between life and death for the experimental animals. In addition, Hopkins demonstrated that the essential unknowns that existed in foods were organic, rather than inorganic, substances that could be dissolved in alcohol.

Work of a similar nature was being carried out at the University of Wisconsin, and at universities in Norway and England.

Research in the field was stimulated greatly in 1912 by a young biologist, Dr. Casimir Funk. He proposed that the then-known dietary deficiency diseases of beriberi, scurvy, pellagra, and rickets were caused by a lack in the diet of special substances that he called *vitamines,* short for *vital amines.* This name caught the popular fancy and has persisted, despite the fact that not all the vital substances turned out to be amines. At the suggestion of J.C. Drummond in 1920, the final e was dropped. Drummond also suggested that the different vitamins be named with the letters of the alphabet, such as A, B, C, D, and E. These changes were quickly accepted.

Vitamins later turned out to be a heterogeneous group of substances that differ widely in their chemical nature and physiological activity.

VITAMIN CLASSIFICATION

Q. *How are vitamins classified?*

A. Vitamins belong to the group of micronutrients. Micronutrients are required by the cells in relatively minute amounts.

A food scientist, skilled in using high-pressure liquid chromatography, is shown separating three types of vitamin B_6 from a model food system.

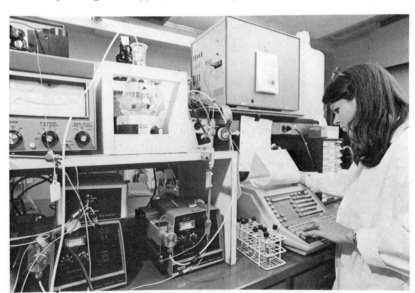

Vitamins can be classified according to whether they are soluble in fat or water. The names that have been accepted are as follows:

Fat-Soluble Vitamins	Water-Soluble Vitamins
Vitamin A	Ascorbic Acid (Vitamin C)
Vitamin D	B-Complex Vitamins
Vitamin E	Thiamin (Vitamin B_1)
Vitamin K	Riboflavin (Vitamin B_2)
	Pyridoxine (Vitamin B_6)
	Nicotinic Acid (Niacin)
	Pantothenic Acid
	Folic Acid
	Vitamin B_{12}
	Biotin

Vitamins occur widely in many foods and are easily provided in a properly prepared mixed diet containing fresh fruits and vegetables. Vitamins are essential because they cannot be synthesized by the body at a sufficient rate to satisfy the body's needs; therefore, they must be present in the diet.

Although the therapeutic effects of vitamin supplementation are very rapid and dramatic in a vitamin-deficient subject, it does not follow that such improvement will occur if the subject had the same symptoms but was not vitamin deficient or if large doses of the vitamin are consumed. That is, such symptoms as lethargy, apathy, loss of appetite, excessive fatigue, and dry or scaly skin may be due to nondietary causes such as infection, insufficient sleep, worry, or other emotional problems.

All the fat-soluble vitamins can be stored to some extent in the body, primarily in the liver. If these vitamins are consumed in excessive amounts, they may accumulate in the body to such an extent that they produce toxic symptoms.

Excess intake of nonstored (water-soluble) vitamins can also produce toxic symptoms.

Although vitamins are often said to "produce energy," they actually cannot. Some of them, however, are necessary as parts of enzyme systems for the release of the energy supplied in the diet by carbohydrates, fats, and proteins.

Q. *Why are vitamins identified by letters and numbers?*
A. At first, no one knew what the substances were chemically. They were identified by letters. Later, what was thought to be one vitamin B turned out to be many, and numbers were added.

Eventually some vitamins were found unnecessary for human needs and were removed from the list, which accounts for some of the gaps in the numbers. These include B_8, adenylic acid, and B_{13}, orotic acid. Vitamins, H, M, S, W, and X were all shown to be biotin. Vitamin G became vitamin B_2, and vitamin Y became B_6. Vitamin M seems to have been used for three different vitamins: folic acid, pantothenic acid, and biotin. The present trend is to eliminate the confusion by using chemical names.

VITAMINS AND ATHLETICS

Q. *Do athletes engaged in rigorous training programs require additional vitamin supplementation?*
A. Athletes who consume large quantities of vitamin pills assume that vitamin requirements are increased during exercise or that it is possible to supercharge the cells of the body by providing them with extra vitamins. Although nutritional articles promoting the use of vitamin supplements by athletes have appeared in a number of magazines under the bylines of well-known physiologists, the arguments remain unconvincing. Furthermore, nutrition scientists have been unable to demonstrate the effectiveness of such nutrient supplements. Vitamin requirements are not increased before or during strenuous exercise, and it is impossible to supercharge the

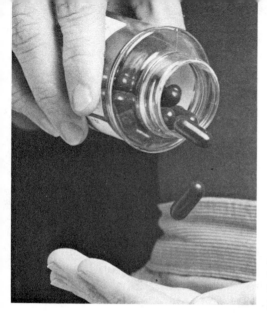

A fitness-minded person who regularly consumes a balanced diet does *not* need to take vitamin pills.

tissue since most vitamins cannot be stored, and any excess amount is rapidly excreted. Extra amounts of the vitamins that can be stored are inactive, of no benefit, or toxic. A healthy athlete ingesting a well-balanced diet receives adequate amounts of all vitamins. The use of vitamin pills without a specific deficiency, therefore, is nothing more than the use of expensive placebos.

Q. *What about all the advertising on television that show various athletes endorsing vitamin supplements?*

A. A typical television commercial shows an athletic-looking man explaining how he stays healthy. He says he watches his diet, gets plenty of exercise, and "just to be sure," takes a daily vitamin supplement. The advertisement implies that a balanced diet cannot provide adequate nutrients. This is untrue. All necessary nutrients are easily obtained from a sensible diet of ordinary foods. The sole exception is that some women who have excessively heavy menstrual periods may need to take iron supplements.

Another type of vitamin advertising will proclaim a relationship to prestigious organizations such as the U.S. Olympic Committee. The USOC will award a company the right to advertise that its product was "selected by" the U.S. Olympic team or that it is "supplier to" or "contributor to" the team.

This is in exchange, of course, for a contribution that helps finance the Olympic athletes' activities. But the advertising that results is not necessarily anything more than a clever inducement to buy the products.

As George V. Mann, M.D., a noted nutritionist and Professor of Biochemistry at the University of Tennessee, commented in *The Physician and Sports Medicine* magazine: "I don't know of any evidence that athletes benefit from supplementary vitamins. . . . The bottom line is that it's pure promotional hyping. This isn't the same thing as an Olympic sweat shirt. Of all the people in the world, international class athletes probably need supplementary vitamins the least."

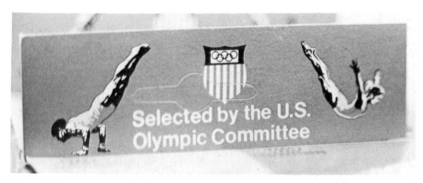

Dr. George V. Mann, a well-known nutritionist interested in sports medicine, cautions people to be aware of the promotional efforts to buy vitamin pills that will precede the 1984 Olympics in Los Angeles. "Of all the people in the world," states Dr. Mann, "international class athletes probably need supplementary vitamins the least."

Q. *Is there any one vitamin that is particularly important to an athlete in training?*

A. All of the 50 or more nutrients work together and are important to an athlete. But there is no particular vitamin or other single nutrient that is uniquely important. From these nutrients the body synthesizes an estimated 10,000 different compounds that are essential to health and performance. A lack of one might result in the underproduction of hundreds

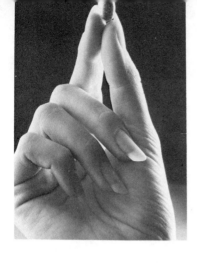

There is *no* single vitamin that is particularly important to the athlete. The four fat-soluble and the nine water-soluble vitamins are all important for maximum performance. Eating a balanced diet will ensure that the athlete gets optimum amounts of all 13 vitamins.

of the essential compounds, but at the same time, adding large amounts of some nutrients may interfere with the functioning of others. The athlete should eat a well-balanced diet composed of a wide variety of foods.

VITAMIN SUPPLEMENTS AND COLD WEATHER

Q. *Do cold weather and increased exercise often associated with winter activities make greater demands on the body for vitamins? If so, is it advisable to take a multivitamin supplement?*

A. The basic need for nutrients is the same in the winter as in the summer. Depending upon the weight of clothing worn, more energy may be needed to keep the body warm when exposure to the cold is extensive, but the average difference between energy needs in warm and cold climates is not great.

There is no need for the athlete to supplement an adequate diet with vitamins during the winter. It has been claimed that large amounts of vitamin C will help prevent flu and the common cold, but no good medical evidence exists to support this claim. Little evidence exists that exercise or heavy work increases vitamin requirements. Increased activity does increase a person's caloric requirements and therefore the requirements for vitamins, thiamin, and niacin, which are involved in energy release. But again, these nutrients will be present in adequate amounts if the diet is balanced.

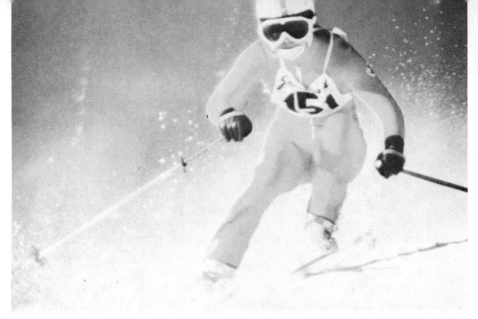

There is no need for an athlete who competes in winter sports, such as snow skiing, to supplement his diet with vitamin pills. (Photo by David Ponsonby)

VITAMIN A IN LARGE DOSES

Q. *Is it harmful to take vitamin A in large quantities, such as 200,000 USP units a day?*

A. The functions of vitamin A relate primarily to eyes and the visual process, to the maintenance of epithelial membranes, and to growth. In addition, vitamin A has sometimes been referred to as the anti-infection vitamin since it does aid in providing satisfactory protective covering and in maintaining part of the body's defense mechanism. But this does not mean that large quantities of vitamin A will improve eyesight or help an individual guard against infection.

At the levels mentioned, an individual would be getting 40 times the recommended allowance for this vitamin. There are only a few abnormal situations in which physicians prescribe special doses of vitamins. Since vitamin A is fat-soluble, large amounts of the vitamin can cause serious tissue damage. If a person has been using large amounts of vitamin A for some time, he would be wise to consult a physician to determine if there have been any adverse effects.

VITAMIN D

Q. *How much vitamin D must be consumed each day? What are the best sources for this vitamin? Is it possible to obtain too much vitamin D?*

A. Vitamin D has an important role in the growth and development of bones and teeth. Consequently, the need for vitamin D is particularly critical during infancy, childhood, pregnancy, and lactation. Vitamin D assists primarily in the absorption of calcium from the intestinal tract into the bloodstream.

The recommended intake of vitamin D for infants and children is 400 USP units per day. This amount of vitamin D will provide for the needs of all infants and children except a very small minority who, because of genetic abnormality, require massive amounts. There is no dietary requirement for vitamin D for adults. A sufficient amount of vitamin precursors are synthesized in the body and converted to the active form in the skin by ultraviolet light when the subject spends a few minutes each day in direct sunlight. A dietary intake of 400 USP units, regardless of sunlight exposure, is generous and entirely adequate. There is, in fact, danger in consuming large amounts of this vitamin since it accumulates in the body and eventually causes toxic symptoms.

Vitamin D may be supplied in our food or generated in the body by exposure to sunlight. (Photo by Ellington Darden)

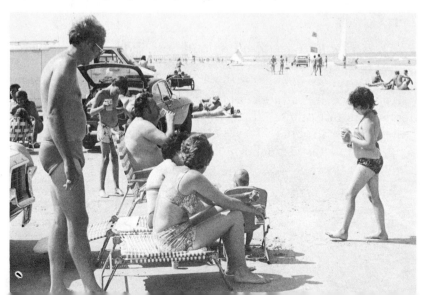

Vitamin D is found in very moderate amounts in a few foods such as eggs, some saltwater fish, and summer milk. Because this vitamin does not occur commonly in nature, it has been standard practice to fortify milk with 400 units of vitamin D per quart. Fluid whole milk, skimmed milk, and evaporated milk have added vitamin D. Most commercial infant formulas are also fortified with vitamin D.

There has been a trend in recent years for some food manufacturers to add vitamin D, along with other vitamins, to various processed foods. The Council of Food and Nutrition of the American Medical Association recommends the fortification of milk and margarine with vitamin D but sees no justification for adding this nutrient to other foods such as breakfast cereals, fruit drinks, and candy. Such an addition of vitamins by the manufacturer is done to sell his products and not to correct a nutritional problem in the safest or best way. The American Academy of Pediatrics estimates that it would not be unusual for a child to consume as many as 2,000 USP units of vitamin D per day from vitamin-fortified foods and supplements. This amounts to more than five times the recommended dietary allowance. A daily intake of 1,800 USP units over prolonged periods of time has been shown to be hazardous to some people.

The tolerance for vitamin D varies with the individual, depending on his endocrine system, his exposure to ultraviolet light, and his dietary intake of calcium.

VITAMIN E

Q. *Is vitamin E required by athletes? What foods are good sources of this vitamin?*

A. Although vitamin E does not have unusual or unique significance for athletic performance, athletes do require a small amount of vitamin E in their diets. Good sources of this vitamin are green leafy vegetables, whole-grain cereals, legumes, and nuts. Smaller amounts of vitamin E are found in eggs and meat.

Q. *Does wheat germ oil, which contains vitamin E, have a beneficial effect on athletic performance, especially endurance-type activities?*

A. Probably more controversy prevails concerning the effects of wheat germ oil and vitamin E on athletic performance than any other supplement. Although wheat germ oil is know to be a potent source of vitamin E and the polyunsaturated fatty acids, the evidence for its value as a nutritional supplement for athletes appears unfounded. Tom Cureton, a physiologist, has reported several nutritional experiments that suggest that wheat germ oil has beneficial effects on the performance of some human subjects in training. But other investigators have not been able to confirm the work of Cureton. A medical team headed by Dr. I. M. Sharman of London found that adolescents receiving wheat germ oil capsules did not differ in performance measures from those of a control group who consumed placebos. Similar findings using college students have recently been reported by John W. Siemann and Dr. Ronald Byrd of Florida State University.

Scientific studies show that wheat germ oil has no positive effect on improving an athlete's endurance.

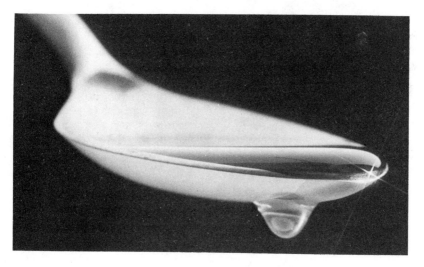

The importance of vitamin E in the human body appears to lie largely in the fact that it is an antioxidant that in some ways affects the oxidation-reduction reactions in the body. Because of this, many athletes in intensive training assume that supplemental vitamin E will improve performance, especially in those events requiring a great deal of endurance. Any apparent beneficial effect of wheat germ oil on the performance of athletes is psychological in nature.

VITAMIN B-COMPLEX

Q. *Many athletes take B-complex and vitamin B_{12} injections in hopes of increasing their strength and energy. Is there any scientific justification for this?*

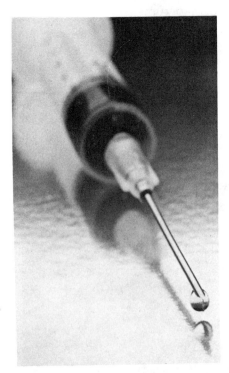

While vitamin B_{12} injections are needed to treat pernicious anemia, they will not produce greater strength or endurance in a healthy athlete.

A. No. There is no reason for a healthy athlete to take B-complex or vitamin B_{12} injections. It is merely a waste of money and the excess vitamins would be excreted in the urine. Someone who feels chronically run down should consult a physican. The cause is unlikely to be dietary.

VITAMIN C AND THE COMMON COLD

Q. *Much has been written about vitamin C and its importance in preventing the common cold. Since a cold can limit performance, should the athlete consume large doses of vitamin C in order to prevent colds?*

A. There is some controversy among medical authorities concerning the use of vitamin C in preventing colds. Most of this controversy involves the recommendations of the chemist, Dr. Linus Pauling, in his book, *Vitamin C and the Common Cold* (1970). Pauling recommends the ingestion of from 1,000 to 5,000 milligrams of vitamin C per day. This is many times over the 60 milligrams per day recommended by the National Research Council.

According to *The Miami Herald*, most of the nutrition experts that were surveyed were doubtful or critical of Dr. Pauling's conclusions. They noted the fact that some people have adverse reactions to massive doses of vitamin C such as diarrhea and the excretion of extraordinary amounts of urine. Dr. Charles Glen King, who originally isolated vitamin C, reports that excessive amounts of this vitamin increase the risk of kidney and bladder stones. Furthermore, there is evidence in the Russian scientific literature that even smaller amounts than those recommended by Pauling are toxic, causing miscarriage in pregnant women. To date, excessive amounts of vitamin C have not been shown to prevent respiratory infections or colds.

Vitamin C does play several important roles in the body. It is involved in the formation and maintenance of bones, periodontal tissues, and teeth. In addition, vitamin C contributes

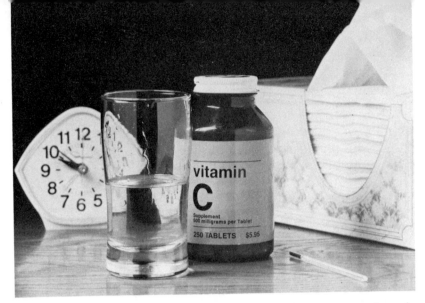

There is no evidence that an intake of vitamin C greater than the recommended dietary allowance will prevent colds.

to wound healing, iron deposits, and the synthesis of adrenal hormones and blood cells. But until more conclusive evidence is available concerning vitamin C and the common cold, the athlete need not consume more vitamin C than the recommended dietary allowance, which can easily be obtained by eating four or more servings of fruits and vegetables or one small glass of fresh or reconstituted orange juice per day.

VITAMIN C AND SMOKING

Q. *What is the relationship between vitamin C requirements and cigarette smoking?*

A. At least three recent studies have reported that the blood concentration of vitamin C is lower in smokers than in nonsmokers. Smokers were found to retain more vitamin C, when large doses were given, than nonsmokers. A study of guinea pigs who were exposed to tobacco smoke also revealed that the vitamin C content of the adrenal glands was reduced. The growth of the guinea pigs also was poorer than that of another group who had not been exposed to smoke. Even more serious, however, is the effect that smoking has on pulmonary function, so important to the performance of all

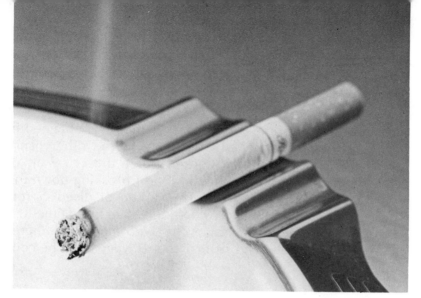

Heavy smokers need slightly more vitamin C than nonsmokers. This need, however, is easily met if the smoker meets the recommended dietary allowance of vitamin C on a daily basis.

body cells and most athletic events. The instant a person inhales cigarette smoke, things begin to happen to the heart, lungs, and body. Smoking starts his heart pounding an extra 15 to 20 beats per minute and raises his blood pressure by 10 to 20 millimeters. In the lungs, smoke chokes the airways and attacks the air sacs, leaving a residue of cancer-causing chemicals. It deposits these and other dangerous poisons in the stomach, kidneys, and bladder. This happens with every cigarette a person smokes. No smoker is immune.

A teenage athlete who smokes may feel winded under mild stress, even if he smokes only five or six cigarettes a day. The smoker will find himself out of breath more quickly than his nonsmoking competitors. Moreover, smokers have a high risk of developing heart disease, lung cancer, and respiratory infections.

RAW VS. COOKED VEGETABLES

Q. *Can athletes obtain more vitamins from raw or cooked vegetables?*

A. The answer to this question depends on the vegetables and the cooking procedures. Vitamin C, found in tomatoes, is water-soluble and heat-labile so cooking washes some of it out and destroys some of it. More vitamin C is obtained in raw tomatoes than cooked tomatoes. On the other hand, vitamin A is fat-soluble and locked inside the cell walls of vegetables. Cooking does a better job of breaking down the cell walls than does chewing. Thus a cup of diced carrots cooked in the correct way provides more than three times the vitamin A of a cup of raw carrots. It is recommended, therefore, that several raw and several cooked vegetables be consumed each day.

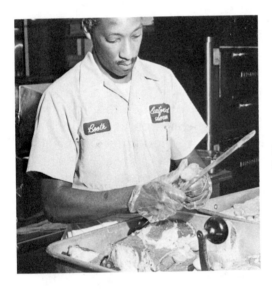

Stewed carrots are an excellent source of vitamin A.

FRESH, FROZEN, OR CANNED

Q. *Are fresh vegetables nutritionally superior to frozen or canned vegetables?*

A. In the industrial canning process, the vegetable is harvested at the proper time to assure optimal size, appearance, and nutritional value. The product is chilled immediately after picking and rushed to the factory. Once at the factory, it is washed and blanched and immediately processed by a short-

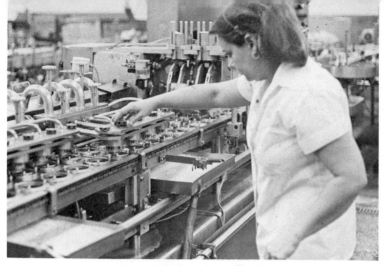

The food preservation techniques in greatest use today do not result in major losses in nutritive value of foods. The more sophisticated methods of food preservation now being developed will retain even higher percentages of nutrients. Above, a portion-packaging machine fills, seals, and quick-freezes orange juice.

term, high-temperature process. This cooking process, followed by a very rapid cooling period, is the key to the superiority of industrial procedures over many home procedures. The vegetable is cooled in a closed system with a minimum amount of air cooking time. If the can is opened at home, it is necessary only to warm the food prior to serving.

In the freezing process, if vegetables are picked and then quick-frozen, the nutrient values are equal to or perhaps even higher than those of fresh vegetables.

Homegrown, freshly harvested vegetables cooked immediately will not usually have greater nutritional value than good-quality processed vegetables. Slow-cooking methods used frequently by homemakers often destroy more vitamins than are lost during the industrial canning process. Conversely, fresh vegetables that have been poorly stored at the market may be less nutritious than those freshly picked from a home garden. Fresh vegetables that are locally grown in season are frequently cheaper than the commercially processed vegetables. But sometimes, even in season, fresh vegetables can be more expensive than canned or frozen ones.

Even though there may be significant loss of nutritive value from vegetables during both industrial and home processing, this loss is more significant to the vegetables than to the consumer. The individual should not be fooled by reports of 10% to 20% nutrient loss unless he knows the amount that remains. Such losses are of little practical significance for anyone who consumes a well-balanced or mixed diet that has not been overcooked and contains some fresh fruits and vegetables each day.

IMPORTANCE OF VEGETABLES

Q. *If all fruits and vegetables are good for athletes, why then are dark green and deep yellow vegetables stressed so much?*

A. Fruits and vegetables that contain similar quantities of nutrients are often combined into general groups in discussing a balanced diet. The dark green and deep yellow vegetables supply important quantities of vitamin A, which is not present in significant quantities in all fruits and vegetables. Furthermore, many of the dark green vegetables can be counted on to provide vitamin C as well as appreciable amounts of iron, riboflavin, calcium, and magnesium.

Nutritionists wishing to emphasize the importance of vegetable sources of vitamin A recommend that a dark green or deep yellow vegetable be eaten at least every other day. Examples of dark green vegetables are spinach, broccoli, kale, collards, and turnip greens. Deep yellow vegetables are carrots, sweet potatoes, squash, and pumpkin.

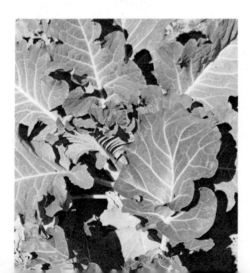

A serving of a green leafy vegetable, such as collards, is a good source of vitamins A, C, and riboflavin.

Certain vegetables and fruits, particularly citrus fruits, are excellent sources of vitamin C. They should be consumed every day to assure an adequate intake of this vitamin. Examples are oranges, grapefruit, cantaloupe, strawberries, and broccoli. The singling out of certain fruits and vegetables should not be interpreted to mean that others are not important. It simply means that such foods are rich sources of certain nutrients.

TRUTH ABOUT VITAMINS

Q. *Concerning vitamin supplements, what is the soundest position for a fitness-minded individual to take?*

A. The fitness-minded individual should remember that he needs vitamins each day. The daily allowances recommended by the National Research Council are established by subcommittees made up of the best experts on each vitamin. These are men and women with research experience with these vitamins in clinical nutrition.

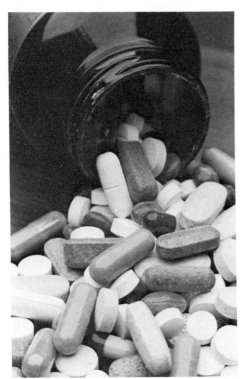

Today, many a misguided customer spends $100 or even $200 a month on special pills, tablets, and capsules to bring vitamins into his life. According to Dr. Thomas Jukes of the University of California's Space Science Laboratory, the bulk wholesale cost of a month's supply of the ten vitamins most frequently found in supplements is less than 6¢. This helps to explain why so many retailers like to sell vitamins.

The allowances contain a generous but reasonable margin of safety to cover individual differences and changing conditions. Large doses much in excess of the allowances are needed only in certain disease states. Under such conditions, vitamin supplements should be prescribed by a physician.

A varied diet with ample amounts of fruits and vegetables, milk, bread, and meat provides more than enough vitamins for the vast majority of Americans. Some individuals with irregular food habits or those on a low-calorie diet may be wise to supplement their daily diet with one vitamin pill containing no more than the recommended daily allowances of all required vitamins. But in all cases the individual's physician should be consulted. As far as megavitamins are concerned, it is important to remember that, in normal amounts, vitamins are food. At 5, 10, 100, or 1,000 times the normal level, vitamins are *drugs* and should be treated accordingly.

8
minerals

DIFFERENCE BETWEEN VITAMINS AND MINERALS

Q. *What is the difference between vitamins and minerals?*

A. Unlike vitamins, minerals tend to be incorporated into the actual structures and working chemicals of the body. Vitamins function mainly as catalysts. They promote chemical processes without actually becoming part of the products of the reactions. Minerals become involved in the building of enzymes and in the building of actual tissue structures.

Much that has been said about vitamins may also be said about minerals. They occur in tiny amounts in foods but evidently in sufficient quantity so that nearly all minerals needed by the body can be found in an ordinary, varied diet. Once the minuscule daily mineral requirements are met, any excess is useless or even toxic.

FUNCTIONS OF MINERALS

Q. *What are the functions of minerals in the human body?*

133

A. Most of the functions that minerals perform in the body may be listed under three main categories: structural, functional, and regulatory components.

As structural components, minerals provide rigidity and strength to bones and teeth.

As functional components, minerals occur in soft tissues and fluids throughout the body, enabling cells to perform many of the functions assigned to them:

1. They help maintain the correct total amount of body fluid as well as its distribution throughout the body.

2. They contribute to the maintenance of a neutral acid-base condition of the blood and body tissues.

3. They make possible normal rhythm of the heartbeat and contractibility of all muscles.

4. They help maintain a normal response of nerves to stimuli.

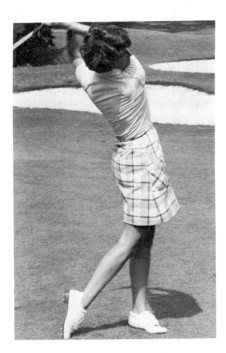

Minerals play an important role in muscular contraction.

5. They are essential for blood clot formation.

As regulatory components, minerals occur as essential parts of many enzymes and hormones that regulate or control most of the body's reactions:

1. Iodine—thyroxine
2. Zinc—insulin
3. Sulfur—vitamin B_1 and biotin
4. Cobalt—vitamin B_{12}
5. Magnesium—enzymes for energy release

Although minerals are identified separately, it should be understood that they act together and in various combinations. While certain minerals serve specific purposes in the body, they rarely act alone in accomplishing these purposes.

MINERAL CLASSIFICATION

Q. *How are minerals classified?*

A. The minerals in the body can be separated into two groups: those that occur in the body and in foods in relatively large amounts and those that occur and are needed in trace amounts. The minerals that occur in large amounts are calcium, phosphorus, magnesium, potassium, sodium chloride, and sulfur. The trace elements are iron, copper, iodine, fluoride, cobalt, manganese, and zinc. The National Research Council has established recommended dietary allowances for calcium, phosphorus, magnesium, iron, iodine, and zinc. It is believed that if the requirements for these and other nutrients on the recommended dietary allowance table are met, then the remaining minerals will also be present in adequate amounts.

MINERALS AND MUSCLE CRAMPS

Q. *Are minerals important in preventing severe muscle cramps that sometimes occur in the legs of cyclists, runners, and football players after extreme physical effort?*

A. Many factors are involved in the physiological responses of muscles during and after prolonged exercise. The tissue content of sodium chloride (table salt) is a critical factor, and this tissue component may be seriously depleted by prolonged physical exercise or perspiration, particularly in hot and humid weather. This depletion can occur even though the athletes have taken what they believed to be adequate quantities of salt before and during exercise. It was reported in a 1971 edition of the *Journal of the American Medical Association*, by Dr. Allan Ryan of the University of Wisconsin, that an athlete may lose as much as three to five grams of salt per liter of sweat. This salt could be replaced by the frequent drinking of salt water (.1–.2% concentrations).

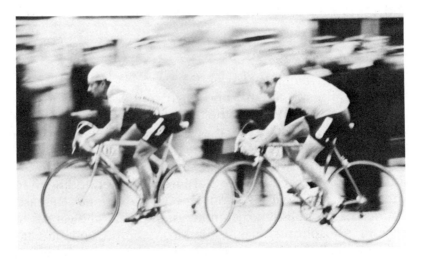

Cyclists often suffer from leg cramps during hot and humid weather. As a preventive measure, large amounts of salt water should be consumed before, during, and after competition. (Photo by David Ponsonby)

Another factor to be considered in leg cramps is the depletion of glycogen in the muscles. The muscle tissues become strongly acidic during vigorous exercise as a result of the accumulation of lactic acid. The normal level for this acid may not be achieved until 24 or more hours after the exercise has been completed. Dr. Ryan therefore recommends that muscle cramps might be prevented by paying more attention to adequate consumption of salt water before the event and ingesting carbohydrate foods and water immediately following the exercise.

CALCIUM FACTS

Q. *Is it true that too much calcium in the diet can cause calcium deposits in the joints?*

A. Calcium is required in the diet throughout life. Suboptimum calcium intake in adults has been indicated recently as a contributing factor in the development of a disease characterized by weakened bones and invalidism. Optimal calcium nutrition should be promoted for athletes, and one of the best sources of calcium is milk or milk products. The recommended amount of milk for adults is one pint per day.

An excessive dietary intake of calcium may cause calcium deposits in the soft tissues of the body, but it will not have any effect on diseases that affect the joints, such as arthritis, gout, and associated conditions. Typically, the protective mechanisms in the body regulate the absorption and output of calcium so that the body retains only a sufficient amount to meet its needs. It should be noted, however, that very excessive intakes of calcium or vitamin D can be detrimental.

Excessive calcium in the diet will not cause calcium deposits in the joints. But this does not mean that a person should consume more than the recommended dietary allowance of calcium each day.

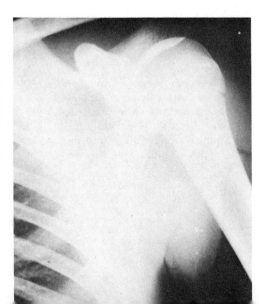

A condition known as hypercalcemia, characterized by excess calcium in the blood, may develop in certain abnormal individuals, in infants, and in young children who have consumed excess vitamin D. Vitamin D aids in calcium absorption in the body and it appears that large amounts of vitamin D can cause an excessive absorption of calcium. This condition can be reversed by decreasing dietary amounts of vitamin D. Hypercalcemia is also found in patients being treated for peptic ulcers with both excessive alkali therapy and excessive milk intake. It does not occur in cases where alkali therapy is not used, even if large amounts of milk are consumed.

Q. *"You never outgrow your need for milk," according to a popular commerical. Is this a correct statement?*

A. According to Dr. Jean Mayer, the statement would be more accurate if it said, "You never outgrow your need for calcium."

While it is true that growing children need more of this essential nutrient than adults, we all require a certain amount of this mineral to carry on a number of vital body functions. Milk is an excellent source of this nutrient as well as others.

Yet there are many people who do not like or cannot drink milk. The person who does not like it can get enough calcium through a wise choice of other foods such as green vegetables, fruits, eggs, and fish. If an individual cannot drink milk

Milk is the most convenient source of calcium. Calcium plays a major role in the structure of bones. The inclusion of a pint of milk daily in the diet of most adults is recommended.

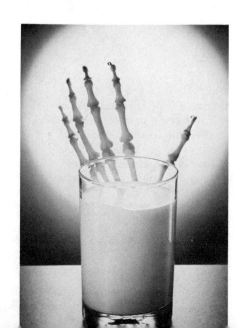

because of an intolerance for lactose, a recent development should help.

An enzyme from yeast put into ordinary milk will split lactose into two simple sugars, glucose and galactose. These simple sugars do not bother lactose-intolerant people.

Small packets of this substance are available at most super-markets. A packet can be added to a quart of milk and can be ready for consumption after overnight refrigeration. People who are lactose-intolerant may want to give it a try.

Lactose is not the cause of every milk allergy, and there are degrees of intolerance. People who believe they are allergic to milk should definitely see a physician.

IMPORTANCE OF FLUORIDE

Q. *If fluoride occurs naturally in foods, why is it necessary to fluoridate public water supplies? What happens to fluoride in the human system?*

A. Much attention has been given to the nutrient fluoride over the past several years, especially as it relates to the fluoridation of the public water supply. Fluoride is a very important nutrient and its deficiency has had a serious effect on the health of many Americans. Small amounts of fluoride are present in most foods. Green plants and seafoods are rich sources, but fluoridated water is the most reliable and certain way of supplying adequate amounts of this nutrient.

Almost all of the body's fluoride (96%) is in the bones and teeth where it represents a storage site that can be called on for use elsewhere in the body when the intake is inadequate.

Flouride is involved in the development of strong bones and teeth. It seems to occupy an essential position in the crystalline structure of these tissues and, if it is not present in adequate amounts, the bones and teeth are weakened.

The evidence for the relationship of fluoride and tooth decay is overwhelming. It is known that the presence of fluoride in enamel, the crown or exposed part of the tooth, makes it a much harder or stronger tissue. Dental decay is

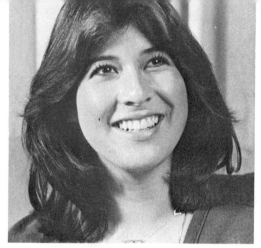

Adequate fluoride is important in the development of strong, attractive teeth. The most reliable source of this essential mineral is fluoridated water at a level of 0.7 to 1.2 parts per million.

reduced 60–70% among children in fluoridated communities. Furthermore, they have fewer missing teeth, less malocclusion, and less periodontal disease. Children whose water supply is not fluoridated should be given fluoride drops or tablets from birth through age 12.

Adequate fluoride nutrition may be shown to have an even more important effect on bone tissue. One of the most debilitating diseases of older age is the weakening of bones, especially among women.

The skeleton or bone tissue is not static once it is laid down. Rather it represents an emergency source of minerals for use by other cells whenever the diet is inadequate. Since such erosion of bone tissue is very slow and occurs without any immediate clinical effects, it may go on for years unnoticed. Unfortunately, the body cannot replace decayed teeth, and once extensive bone erosion and fracture have occurred, healing is almost nonexistent.

IRON

Q. *Since so many iron-fortified foods are on the market, is there a shortage of iron in the American diet?*

A. Iron is an important constituent of blood hemoglobin. Iron reserves in women are important as a protection against iron depletion when blood is lost during menses and childbirth. Extra iron is also needed during pregnancy and lactation. The amount of dietary iron absorbed from food varies according to need. It is this increased dietary absorption, coupled with adequate body iron reserves, that affords protection against the consequences of iron loss or increased need for iron.

A deficiency of iron in the body may express itself as an anemia that is characterized by a subnormal amount of iron or hemoglobin in the blood. An anemic person may be weak, listless, and have unjustified fatigue, loss of appetite, retarded growth, and reduced resistance to disease. Recent surveys indicate that most adolescent boys consume adequate amounts of iron. Nutritionists and blood specialists, however, are concerned by reports that young girls and women consume diets that provide only about half of their iron requirements. The American Medical Association and the National Research Council recommend a daily intake of at least 18 to 20 milligrams of iron for women who menstruate. But studies have found that these women, who have a greater need for iron than men, consume an average of 8 to 10 milligrams per day. Women should be encouraged to eat iron-fortified foods as well as iron-rich foods such as meat, eggs, green vegetables, and whole-grain and enriched cereals. Furthermore, women who are thinking about starting a family should be sure they have adequate body stores of iron to see them through their pregnancies.

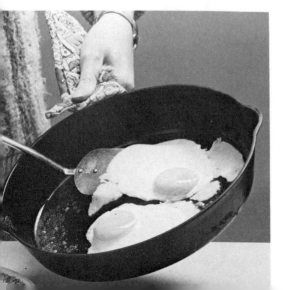

Knowledgeable cooking can enhance the amount of iron delivered by the diet. The iron content of eggs, for example, can be tripled by cooking them in an unenameled iron skillet.

ZINC

Q. *Much is being written about zinc in human nutrition. How important is zinc?*

A. Zinc plays a fundamental role in growth, development, tissue repair, and appetite regulation. Human disorders responsive to zinc supplementation include hypogonadism, growth retardation, impaired wound healing, and diminished taste acuity. Zinc serves as a component of several key enzymes and helps maintain the structural configuration of molecules and membranes.

An adequate zinc intake is of particular importance during pregnancy and other periods of rapid growth and development. The loss of large amounts of body zinc during periods of weight loss contributes to the risk of zinc deficiency in our weight-loss society. Stresses associated with menopause and aging may bring about an increased zinc requirement.

As in the case of several other nutrients, human beings are apparently able to adapt to a fairly wide range of zinc intake from either plant or animal sources. Oysters and red meats are among the richest sources of zinc. Substantial amounts of zinc are also present in whole-grain cereals and legumes. Severe deficiencies of zinc, calcium, and iron often occur in populations subsisting on large amounts of unleavened bread made from whole wheat and bran. Prolonged intakes of such high-fiber diets interfere with the gastrointestinal absorption of these minerals.

MINERAL SUPPLEMENTS

Q. *Wouldn't it be easier for a fitness-minded person simply to consume mineral pills each day than to be so concerned with eating a wide variety of mineral-rich foods?*

A. Granted, it might be easier to take mineral pills than eat a wide variety of foods. One pill a day, however, often can lead to two pills a day—then four, eight, and finally megadoses. It has been proved that all minerals are toxic if taken in excessive amounts.

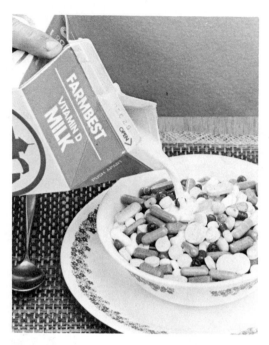

Many athletes assume that if a little bit of each essential mineral is required for good health, then larger amounts of each mineral can produce superhealth. This is not true. In fact, nutritional research shows that all minerals are toxic if taken in excessive amounts.

If the daily requirement of potassium is taken in a single supplemental dose, it can be fatal for certain types of patients. Similarly, smaller supplements taken over a period of time can cause severe ulceration and perforation of the gastrointestinal tract.

The effect of different minerals varies greatly and is influenced by such factors as the individual's state of health, the form in which they are taken, and the levels of other essential minerals and nutrients in the body. While considerable research remains to be done, here are a few things a person should remember.

The effect of calcium depends on its relationship to vitamin D, phosphorus, protein, zinc, lactose, fat, and oxalic and phytic acids. Thus, very high intakes can cause kidney stones or calcium deposits in soft tissues and also increase the severity of zinc and magnesium deficiencies.

Two to five times the normal daily intake of magnesium is a

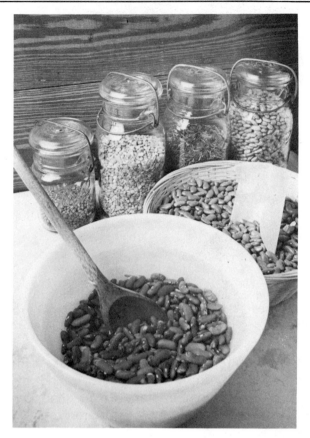

Peas and beans are excellent sources of many essential minerals.

strong bowel stimulant, and larger amounts can lead to death.

An excess of phosphorus over calcium intake interferes with calcium absorption and can bring on mineral loss from the bones, or osteoporosis, in older people.

If an individual is still bound and determined to consume these pills, then the safe course is to buy only the supplements that provide no more than the Recommended Daily Allowance and that are made by reputable manufacturers. And, above all, he should not take supplements without the advice of a physician or registered dietitian.

9

water

IMPORTANCE OF WATER

Q. *Why is water important?*

A. Water is an essential nutrient even though it is often ignored when the nutritional needs of the body are discussed. The body's need for water is exceeded only by that for oxygen. The length of time an individual can do without water depends on the environment. In the middle of the desert on a hot day, a person might remain alive less than 10 hours, while he might remain alive for several days in a more favorable environment. On the other hand, individuals have gone without food for long periods of time and survived, provided they had access to adequate amounts of water.

Approximately 65% of body weight is composed of water. The total water volume is related to the mass of lean tissues of the body rather than to body weight, as fat tissue contains less water than lean tissue. Two-thirds of the body's water is contained within the cells and the remaining one-third is found in spaces outside the cells. Somewhere between three and four quarts of water as blood are constantly circulated to every cell in the body.

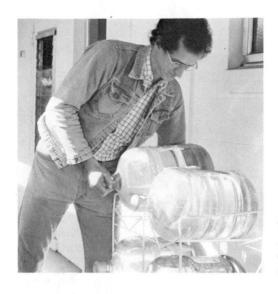

The amount of water in an average man's body is enough to fill two five-gallon bottles.

FUNCTIONS OF WATER

Q. *What are the functions of water inside the human body?*

A. Water functions in the body as a building material, solvent, lubricant, and temperature regulator. It serves as a building material in the construction of every cell and the different cells vary in their water content. The water content of some tissues is as follows: teeth—less than 10%; bone—25%; striated muscle—70%.

As a solvent, water is used in the digestive processes where it aids the chewing and softening of food. It also supplies fluid for the digestive juices and facilitates the movement of the food mass along the digestive tract. After digestion, water as blood is the means by which the nutrients are carried to the cells and waste products are removed.

Water also serves as a lubricant in the joints and between internal organs. As a lubricant, it keeps body cells moist and permits the passage of substances between the cells and blood vessels. Water also plays the very important function of removing heat from the body by its evaporation as sweat.

Q. *How is water distributed in the body?*

A. Water within the body is distributed among several distinct compartments. Approximately 60% of the total body water is found within the cells and is called intracellular fluid. Within each cell the water is subdivided into yet smaller compartments. The other 40% of the total body water is called extracellular fluid. Most of the extracellular fluid surrounds and bathes the cells. Less than 20% of the extracellular fluid is in the blood. Bones, joints, and hollow organs also contain extracellular fluid.

COMPOSITION OF BODY FLUIDS

Q. *What is the composition of body fluids?*

A. The major mineral elements present in body fluids are known as *electrolytes*. The sodium and chlorine (as chloride) content of extracellular fluid is equivalent to a 0.9% solution of common table salt. Smaller amounts of potassium, calcium, magnesium, phosphorus, and sulfur are also present. The fluid inside the cell is very high in potassium and phosphorus. It also contains more magnesium, sulfur, and protein than the extracellular fluids. Measuring the amount of radioactive potassium naturally present in the body is one method of estimating the amount of lean tissue in a living person. Under the influence of electrolytes, such as sodium and potassium, fluid moves continuously in and out of cells carrying oxygen, nutrients, and other chemicals.

MAINTENANCE OF BODY WATER

Q. *How is body water balance maintained?*

A. The kidneys play a key role in maintaining body water balance. Any excess water is readily excreted. Urine becomes more concentrated and less water is excreted by the kidneys when fluid intake is limited.

If, for any reason, excessive sodium is retained by the body, more water is also retained to dilute it and the volume of the extracellular fluid increases. Abnormally large amounts of water surrounding the body's cells cause edema or swelling.

This may occur under certain hormonal influences or in kidney, heart, or liver disease. If the kidneys are not functioning properly, water accumulates and complications of high blood pressure and heart failure may occur.

WATER CONTENT OF FOODS

Q. *Which foods contain water?*

A. Water for the body comes from several sources: beverages and liquids of the diet, water contained in the solid foods of the diet, and water produced by the metabolism of the energy nutrients within the tissues. Naturally, the largest amount of body water comes from ingested beverages such as water, coffee, tea, milk, and fruit juices. Many solid foods in the diet contain more then 70% water. The table on page 149 indicates the percentage of water in some common foods.

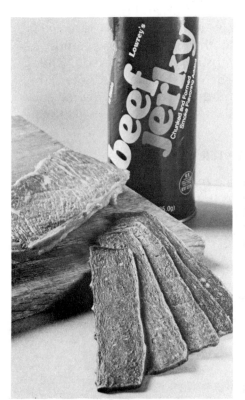

One of the best ways to preserve foods is dehydration. When lean beef is dehydrated, it is reduced to less than 50% of its original size and becomes beef jerky.

Average Water Content of Typical Foods

1.	Lettuce	96%
2.	Celery	94%
3.	Watermelon	93%
4.	Beans, green snap	92%
5.	Broccoli	91%
6.	Apples, raw	85%
7.	Potatoes, white	80%
8.	Bananas	76%
9.	Beef, round, cooked	55%
10.	Bread, white	36%
11.	Butter	16%
12.	Crackers, soda	4%

Water is produced as a by-product whenever carbohydrates, fats, and proteins are utilized in the body. The amount of water produced by different food substances varies according to the following estimated scales:

1 gram of carbohydrate = 0.6 grams of water
1 gram of fat = 1.07 grams of water
1 gram of protein = 0.41 grams of water

REQUIREMENTS FOR WATER

Q. *How much water should a person drink each day?*
A. For the young adult and athlete, activity and environmental conditions are the two most important factors that determine the body's need for water. During study, rest, and sleep, the loss of water from the body is much less than it is during active exercise such as tennis, soccer, and football. When the temperature is hot and humidity low, more water evaporates from the body surface. In most individuals, thirst or the desire for water is an adequate signal of the needs of the body. In certain situations where extreme sweating takes place, or where the air is very dry, the thirst mechanism may

not allow for the drinking of enough water. In these cases it becomes necessary to increase the intake of fluids. Generally speaking, five or six glasses of liquid should be consumed daily by the sedentary individual. Since so many factors affect the requirement for water, however, there is no single figure that would represent the requirement for all people of a given age or sex. The National Research Council states that a reasonable standard for calculating the daily water allowances is one milliliter per calorie of food.

WATER AND ATHLETIC COMPETITION

Q. *If an athlete drinks water during competition, will this be harmful or detrimental to his performance?*

A. Some people think it is harmful to drink water during physical activity. They argue that if an athlete drank all the water he wanted, he would not perform at his maximum. Although this might be true immediately after the intake when the stomach is distended, or when the bladder is full, scientific evidence generally does not support any detrimental long-term effect. Excessive water losses through sweat frequently cause mental confusion, which could definitely affect an athlete's performance. More athletes have probably been affected by too little water intake during performance than too much. The athlete should be allowed to drink as much water as he wishes.

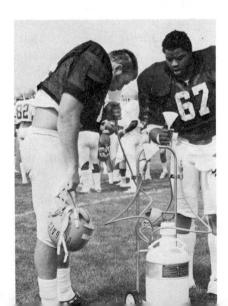

Athletes should be allowed to drink unlimited amounts of water during practice or competition. (Photo by Ellington Darden)

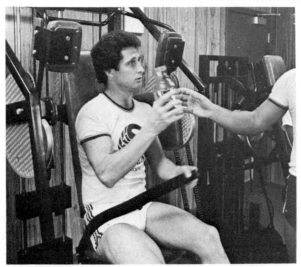

A trainee involved in a high-intensity Nautilus workout should drink water frequently between exercises.

DRINKING WATER DURING NAUTILUS WORKOUTS

Q. *What about drinking water during a Nautilus workout?
Is this recommended?*

A. A Nautilus trainee should be allowed to drink water
any time he desires it. Of course, much of the thirst mechanism is directly related to the temperature and humidity of
the workout room and the intensity of the exercise. A good
rule of thumb is for the trainee to drink several ounces of
water prior to going into the workout area. Another drink is
taken after he completes the lower body machines. More
water can be consumed after the torso machines are finished,
and again when the final machine is completed.

Drinking water, however, can present a problem if a trainee
desires to get his heart rate up to a certain level, such as 150
beats per minute, and keep it there for the duration of the
workout. Rather than hurry back and forth between machines
and the water fountain, he may want to have a bottle of water
placed next to certain machines. The flow of people in the

training area and the rules and regulations of the fitness center also must be considered. Usually, however, compromises can be made to suit everybody's needs.

SWEATING AND PHYSICAL FITNESS

Q. *What does sweating have to do with physical fitness?*

A. While exercising, heat is produced in proportion to the amount of muscle activity. The body's temperature could easily rise as much as 10 degrees or more if this heat were not dissipated. Fortunately, the body is designed to keep itself from overheating. Warm blood is brought to the skin where it loses heat to the surrounding air. The sweat glands begin to secrete water and the body is further cooled by evaporation of the perspiration. In cold weather heat is given off easily. But in hot weather the body must sweat profusely in order to cool itself.

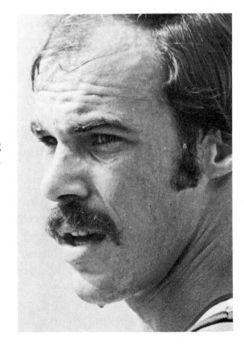

The primary function of sweating is to lower body temperature. (Photo by Inge Cook)

Sweating does not help a person reduce body fat. He may weigh less after a workout, but this is due to a loss of water, not fat. As soon as he quenches his thirst, he will gain the weight back.

Sweating does not clean out the pores. There is no evidence that it is of any value in removing toxic materials from the body. In this respect, an individual should particularly avoid the rubber sweat suits, belts, and wraps. Even steam and sauna baths can lead to problems rather than fitness.

Sweating does not promote fitness. Fitness is developed by exercising the muscles of the body, not the sweat glands.

HEAT VS. HUMIDITY

Q. *Is heat or humidity the bigger problem in dehydration?*

A. Humidity is the bigger problem. On a humid day, evaporation of sweat is hindered because the air, already saturated with its own moisture, has more difficulty absorbing the moisture from a sweating athlete. The body remains encased in its heat envelope, and the blood, with the natural lubrication of body fluids already gone to sweat, thickens. The heart has to take up the slack, pumping harder just to keep up with the same workload.

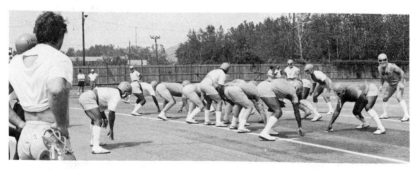

During hot weather practice, as much skin as possible should be exposed to the air. The football players in the above photograph could improve the body's cooling mechanism by wearing shorter socks. (Photo by Ellington Darden)

Athletes such as football players must consider other factors as well. Tight, heavy uniforms and equipment can compound the heat and humidity. This is why many teams wear net jerseys, no T-shirts, light-colored pants, and no high-top stockings.

When profuse sweating does occur, the athlete must stay hydrated as much as possible. This means that large amounts of fluid should be consumed before, during, and after training.

HEAT ILLNESS

Q. *What happens to an athlete who does not cool off and does not drink enough water?*

A. Heat illness is the result. All athletes, therefore, should have a basic understanding of the four types of heat illness:

1. *Heat cramps*—depletion of minerals.

2. *Heat fatigue*—depletion of minerals and water due to excessive fatigue.

3. *Heat exhaustion*—severe depletion of minerals and water.

4. *Heat stroke*—severe dehydration resulting in overheating from breakdown of the sweating mechanism.

Muscular cramps in the thighs and calves are one of the first signs of mineral and water depletion. Immediate care should be given in the form of rest, water, and cooling. (Photo by Ellington Darden)

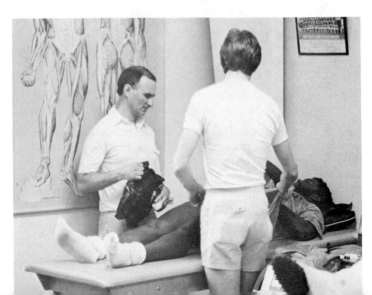

Heat cramps are only temporary, but their moment of occurrence may be disabling. Heat fatigue gradually saps the athlete's strength and dulls his alertness. This decreases his performance capabilities and makes him more vulnerable to injury. Although heat exhaustion and heat stroke can result in serious harm or death, both are preventable.

PREVENTION OF HEAT ILLNESS

Q. *How can heat illness be prevented?*

A. The following precautions are recommended to help athletes prevent heat illness:

1. Become acclimated to hot-weather activity gradually.

2. Schedule training or practice sessions during cooler morning and early evening hours.

3. Take frequent rest periods during practice sessions—at least 15 minutes every hour.

4. Drink ice cold liquids during rest periods. Water is best. Six ounces can be consumed every 15 minutes.

5. Consume large amounts of fluids before and after practice.

6. Keep accurate records of body weight before and after practice sessions. Athletes who lose three percent of their body weight should be observed carefully and forced to drink fluids. Six percent or more weight loss can lead to heat stroke.

7. Do not consume salt tablets. If extra salt is needed, the athlete should use more salt on his food.

8. Wear brief, light-colored clothing. Rubberized apparel should be avoided during hot weather.

9. Become as lean as possible. Subcutaneous fat acts as an insulator.

10. Be conscious of temperature and humidity during practice. The simplest method of measuring the danger of a hot day is with a combination wet and dry bulb thermometer.

11. Watch for signs of lethargy, personality change, stupor, awkwardness, or unusual fatigue.

12. Know what to do in an emergency. Learn the imme-

diate first aid practices and prearrange procedures for obtaining medical care. The onset of heat stroke presents little time for decision making.

DANGERS OF STEAM AND SAUNA BATHS

Q. *Many fitness centers have steam rooms. Why are they dangerous?*

A. One of the biggest dangers connected with steam rooms is the exposure to extreme heat and humidity. Everyone complains when the summer temperature rises to 95 degrees with the humidity close to 100%. Yet, a steam room offers higher temperatures with 100% humidity. Because of the very high humidity, sweat cannot evaporate and cool the body. It is important to recall that the purpose of sweat is to cool the body. Without this cooling effect, body temperature can rise to dangerous levels.

SAUNA BATHS

Q. *Is taking a sauna bath better for a person than taking a steam bath?*

A. Forced to decide between the two, a fitness-minded person would be wise to choose the sauna. The reason is that the humidity is low, which allows the person's sweat to evaporate for maintenance of body temperature. But once again, there is no inherent value in sweating. Sweating alone will not improve a person's level of fitness.

Q. *But won't a sauna bath help eliminate body poisons?*

A. There is absolutely no research to prove that sweating eliminates poisons from the body. The body is neither detoxified nor cleaned by excessive perspiration. Excessive sweating, in fact, causes a tremendous loss of water and electrolytes, which can have a harmful effect on the body.

CHERYL AND THE SCALES:
How Not to Lose Five Pounds in a Day

Cheryl is a thirty-year-old housewife with two children. She is happily married but has one annoying problem. She is getting fat and out of shape.

When the scales registered 140 pounds, she made up her mind to do something about that fat. She had not played tennis in several years. Acting on the determination to lose that fat, she went to the tennis court and played for three hours in the broiling sun. She skipped lunch and took a sauna bath until she almost dropped from exhaustion.

Staggering out of the sauna bath, she got on the scales. To her delight she had lost five pounds.

That evening, she had guests for dinner. With the cocktails, the trout amandine, all the extra dishes, and a rich dessert, Cheryl's dinner was high in both calories and fluid. When her guests left, she got on the scales. To her horror, the scales read, not 135, not 140, but 142 pounds.

What happened to the five pounds Cheryl had lost that afternoon?

Weak after the sauna, she drank two glasses of water. At home, she drank a large ginger ale while helping the maid prepare dinner for her guests. Before dinner, she joined her friends in several cocktails. Along with the four-course meal she drank two glasses of wine and another glass of water. Her total food and drink intake was approximately 112 ounces, or seven pounds.

At the tennis court and in the sauna, Cheryl had lost five pounds of water from sweat. None of this water came from her stored fat. All the liquid she drank, along with the food at the dinner party, not only replaced but increased the fluid she had lost on the tennis court and in the sauna.

Cheryl intended to lose fat, but all she lost was weight in the form of sweat. The total number of calories she consumed for the day was 2,650. Her total caloric expenditure was 2,550. She came out with 100 surplus calories and added 1/35 of a pound to her other fat.

One pint of water weighs one pound. A gallon of water weighs eight pounds. An overweight person can lose four or five pounds from sweat on a hot afternoon or in a sauna bath. Fluid loss has to be replaced. Nature forces the body through thirst to return to its fluid equilibrium.

There is only one way to lose fat: expend more calories than are consumed. Fat loss and weight loss are two different processes. Weight can be lost quickly. Fat cannot.

—Dr. Ellington Darden
From *The Complete Encyclopedia of Weight Loss, Body Shaping and Slenderizing*

Q. *What about using a sauna to relieve muscle aches and pains?*

A. According to Dr. Charles Kuntzleman, national YMCA fitness consultant, muscle aches and pains are difficult to evaluate. If they are caused by muscular or nervous tension, it is possible that a sauna may relax the muscles or tranquilize the nervous system. But whether or not such a treatment would relieve aches and pains has not been confirmed by research. The great majority of the claims made for the sauna are high in personal testimony but thin in research.

SAUNA GUIDELINES

Q. *Some people like to take a sauna because they like the feel of it. Are there any safety guidelines to follow?*

A. It cannot be emphasized too often that a sauna should not be regarded as a means to achieve physical fitness. Those who choose to use the sauna, however, should adhere strictly to the following guidelines:

1. Do not go into a sauna immediately after a high-intensity workout. Cool down first. Or better yet, take a sauna *before* a workout. In this manner, it becomes an effective warm-up.

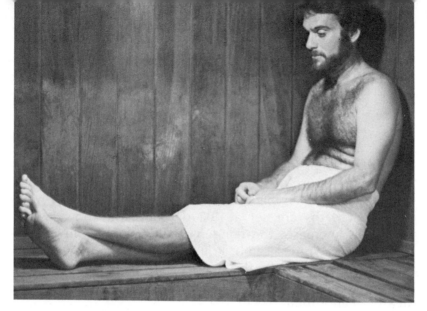

Sweating in a sauna bath will *not* improve an individual's level of fitness.

2. Check to make certain the temperature is no higher than 185 degrees Fahrenheit. The humidity should be at about 10%.

3. Wear as little clothing as possible.

4. Spend no longer than 8 to 10 minutes in the sauna and be sure there is another person in attendance.

5. Do not go into a sauna with a full stomach. Wait at least two hours.

6. Do not use a sauna under the influence of alcohol or narcotics or when antihistamines, tranquilizers, vasoconstrictors, vasodilators, or stimulants have been taken.

7. Do not use a sauna if suffering from diabetes, heart disease, or high blood pressure. Elderly people would be wise to avoid saunas altogether.

WHIRLPOOL BATHS

Q. *What about using whirlpool baths?*

A. Physicians and therapists often recommend whirlpool therapy for people with certain muscle, tendon, and ligament injuries. From a physical fitness rather than rehabilitation viewpoint, however, there are no beneficial effects from soaking in a whirlpool. There are, in fact, several good reasons why a fitness-minded person should avoid using a whirlpool.

First is the problem of heat dissipation. Once a person's body temperature rises above 100 degrees Fahrenheit, serious things begin to happen. The temperature gauges on many whirlpool baths are set at 102 degrees and above, which drastically increases the danger of a person fainting in the water. Dr. Lawrence Lamb, editor of *The Health Letter,* says there is no reason why the temperature of the water should be in excess of body temperature, specifically, above 98 degrees Fahrenheit.

Second, there is a danger of infection from unsanitary water. Warm water has a stimulating effect on the urinary bladder and we all know what usually results. Infection can spread from fecal matter, genital problems, boils, open sores, and wounds. Furthermore, the warm water of a whirlpool makes an excellent breeding environment for many bacteria. Realizing these facts, physical therapists who use whirlpools in their rehabilitation work are careful to drain the water and scrub the tub after each patient uses it. In contrast, the procedure in many fitness centers is to clean the whirlpool nightly and to drain and replace water weekly. This is something to be aware of.

WATER WITH MEALS

Q. *Is there any truth to the common concept of "eat first, drink later"?*

A. Whether the liquid is water or another beverage, it is not harmful to drink during a meal. It is a bad habit, however, to use excessive amounts of liquid to wash food down without chewing it well. But even then, the digestive juices are usually sufficiently powerful to handle most large pieces of food. Drinking a large volume of beverage just prior to eating could cause distension or give an uncomfortable feeling of fullness and thereby reduce the appetite. Beverages that are cold or iced should be drunk more slowly because, if they are consumed quickly, normal stomach functioning may be interrupted. Common sense, therefore, should be used by the athlete when it comes to drinking liquids with meals.

THIRST QUENCHERS

Q. *What is the value of the action drinks promoted for athletes and other extremely active people?*

A. The action drinks include several products new to the beverage market. These products have been referred to as sports drinks, thirst quenchers, oral electrolyte mixtures, and perhaps other terms. Actually, they are diluted solutions of glucose, potassium, sodium chloride and other salts, citric acid, and an artificial sweetener. Although the action drinks were originally prepared for athletes, the manufacturers have broadened their promotions to include all individuals who work hard, play hard, or just get thirsty. And for wider appeal, the beverages now come in several flavors. At least one brand is carbonated and at least one brand has vitamin C added.

These action drinks were designed to serve as thirst-satisfying means of replacing electrolytes and water lost in perspiration. One study suggested that the electrolyte solution is much more rapidly absorbed than water. Also, depending on the brand, 200 to 300 calories may be supplied from the sugar in a quart.

The minerals other than sodium and potassium found in action drinks are not thought to be of any value. As for

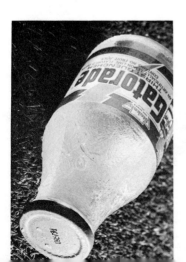

Gatorade was originally formulated by Dr. Robert Cade for the football team at the University of Florida. In choosing a thirst-quenching drink, Dr. Cade says that the athlete should make sure it lists potassium on the label.

sodium, approximately a quart of the beverage must be consumed to supply the equivalent of one gram of salt. If sweating is mild to moderate, the sodium provided by the normal intake of salt in the diet is sufficient. Furthermore, if a person sweats heavily and often, he should be certain to consume potassium-rich foods each day or choose an action drink that contains potassium.

An individual can make an action drink, or saline solution, at home for about one-tenth the cost of the commercially available product. All that is needed is a quart of water, ½ teaspoon of iodized salt, plus a little sugar and flavoring.

COFFEE, TEA, COLA, AND CAFFEINE

Q. *Are coffee, tea, and cola beverages harmful to athletes because of their caffeine content?*

A. Tolerance to caffeine varies widely among individuals. A normal person can tolerate the amount of caffeine in most beverages without apparent discomfort. However, those with such illnesses as active peptic ulcer, hypertension, heart disease, and nervous disorders usually must restrict their intake of products containing caffeine because of the stimulating effect. There is no evidence to show that small amounts of these beverages are harmful in a training diet. On the other hand, there is a good reason for the athlete to avoid them just before an event. Coffee, tea, and cola, while stimulants, may have a depressing effect on the athletes three or four hours later and possibly impair performance if consumed at the meal preceding exercise.

Coffee is still the most popular beverage for many adults in the United States.

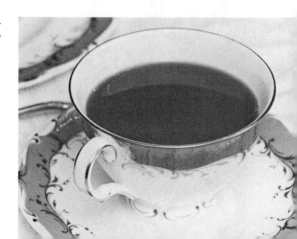

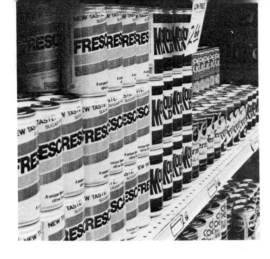

Soft drinks consist of 86 to 93% purified water and up to 14% sugar.

A five-ounce cup of coffee, prepared from 15 to 17 grams of coffee, contains about 18 milligrams of caffeine per fluid ounce or a total of 90 milligrams. The caffeine of coffee, among other effects on the nervous system, may cause sleeplessness in some people. A cup of tea contains approximately 12 to 15 milligrams of a related stimulant per fluid ounce or 60 to 75 milligrams per cup. Cola drinks contain caffeine in amounts ranging from 18 to 28 milligrams for a six-ounce bottle of cola.

BOTTLED WATERS

Q. *What about the current rage over bottled waters?*

A. The initial rage over water got its start more than 50 years ago. Presidents, movie stars, and members of high society flocked to places famed for their water—Calistoga in California, Saratoga in New York, Poland Spring in Maine, and Hot Springs in Arkansas. This rage, however, did not catch on with the masses. Only a few small companies in the United States distributed bottled water.

But the popularity of bottled water began to grow in 1977. Great Waters of France, which sells Perrier, found that people would pay $4 to $5 a gallon for water. Perrier, through clever advertising, began to appeal to people's desire to be glamorous, sophisticated, and rich. In addition, Perrier and other bottled waters as well, began to use words in their advertising such as "natural," "no calories," and "health." It must have worked, because Perrier sales zoomed from about 3 million bottles in 1976 to an estimated 200 million bottles in 1979.

Evidently, the bottled water business has evolved to the point where it is not an alternative to tap water, but an alternative to soft drinks and alcoholic beverages. Twenty-five cents for a glass of water may not seem so expensive after all.

Q. *Is there anything special about various bottled waters?*

A. The only thing special about bottled waters is the cost, which can range from several cents to 36¢ per eight-ounce serving. Plain tap water, on the other hand, costs virtually nothing. A close look at some bottled waters should prove helpful.

Since water is a universal solvent, it can contain dissolved gases such as carbon dioxide and minerals such as calcium, iron, and salt compounds. Solid matter can be suspended in it as tiny particles and bacteria and other microorganisms can live in it.

In 1980 Consumers Union, which publishes *Consumer Reports*, tested and evaluated 38 kinds of water.* Twenty-three of the waters were the sparkling or carbonated kind and 15 were still waters without gas bubbles.

One measurement that Consumers Union used is called "total dissolved solids." Total dissolved solids has become an important measurement in the official definition of mineral water. In California, for example, if a bottled water has 500 parts per million (ppm) or more of total dissolved solids, it must be labeled as a "mineral water." With less than 500 ppm, it cannot be labeled as such. Perrier, under the regulation, tested out at 545 ppm, Canada Dry Club Soda measured 536, and Poland Spring Sparkling a mere 99 ppm. The last two are

---

*Copyright 1980 by Consumers Union of United States, Inc., Mount Vernon, NY 10550. Excerpted by permission from *Consumer Reports*, September 1980.

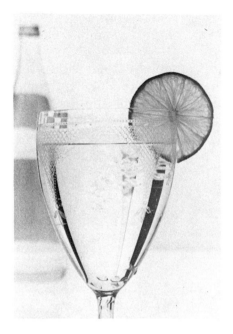

The bottled water business has evolved to the point that it is an alternative to soft drinks and alcoholic beverages. Even so, chemical analyses show that the only thing special about bottled water is the cost.

of particular interest because Poland Spring's label claims it to be a mineral water, which it is not, and Canada Dry Club Soda's label does not claim to be a mineral water, which it is.

The amount of dissolved solids, mostly calcium and magnesium compounds, also determines whether a water is hard or soft. Generally, the more minerals, the harder the water. New York City's tap water is naturally soft at 60 ppm. Other waters, such as Vichy Celestinos and Calso, had high levels of minerals, 3,400 ppm and 5,100 ppm respectively. (After publication date of the Consumers Union study, Calso changed in mineral content. As of February 19, 1981, it measured 3,255 ppm.)

Blind-testing the waters according to taste, under strictly controlled conditions, revealed interesting conclusions. Consumers Union's sensory consultants judged New York City's tap water excellent along with two other still waters. It is humorous that this ordinary tap water, at a cost of next to nothing, was declared by expert tasters as "everything an excellent water should be." The experts also considered Deep Rock Artesian-Fresh Drinking Water and Mountain Valley to be of similar quality.

Where sparkling waters are concerned, the water should be free of any strong or lingering flavors. It should look and taste bubbly. The expert tasters judged none of the sparkling waters excellent. None was rated very good. Perrier and Canada Dry Club Soda, the two big sellers among the sparkling waters, were considered mildly bitter and salty.

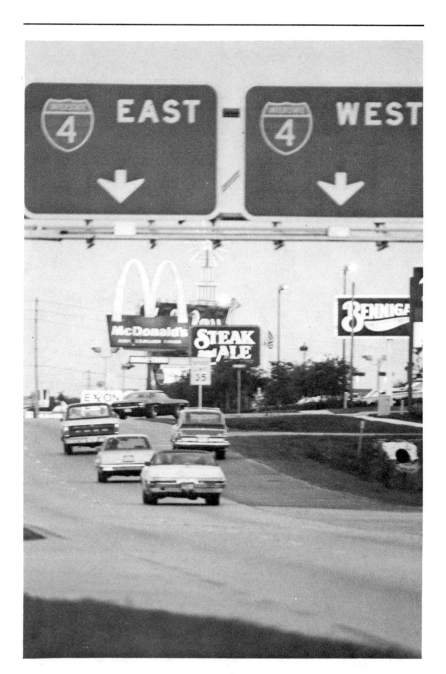

III.

CONTROVERSIAL FOODS

10

---

sugar

SUGAR DEFINED

Q. *What is sugar?*

A. Sugars are the basic form of carbohydrate. They are widespread throughout nature, occurring in fruits, vegetables, nectar, honey, blood, milk, and as building blocks of simple and complex organic molecules. The simple sugars, glucose and fructose, are found in virtually all plants, separately and in combination.

Our major source of sugar is sucrose. This is the familiar refined white sugar, obtained from cane or beets, which is commonly added to our food. Sucrose is formed when a molecule of glucose combines with a molecule of fructose.

COMPARISON OF SUGARS

Q. *Is there any truth to the idea that one sugar is somehow better than another?*

A. A quick walk through a health food store may suggest that white sugar is rated on par with DDT and arsenic. But

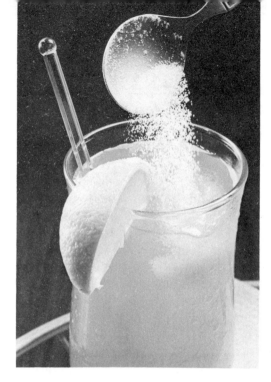

Common table sugar (sucrose) is a sweet crystallizable material obtained commercially from sugar cane or sugar beets. It contains 15 calories per teaspoon.

that does not mean that sugar is eliminated in their products. The breads, for example, are full of honey, brown sugar, or raw sugar. Only white refined sugar is considered the villain.

Nutritionally, however, there is virtually no difference among the various types of sugars. To understand why, let us examine how sucrose is made.

In a typical manufacturing operation, sugar cane is shredded into small pieces, crushed, and the juice separated. Processing causes the sugar in the juice to crystallize, forming sugar crystals and syrup. These are separated by a mechanical device into raw sugar and molasses. A washing and filtering process soon turns the raw sugar into a refined white sugar.

Real raw sugar cannot be sold in the United States because it contains contaminants such as insect parts, soil, molds, bacteria, lint, and waxes. When it is partially refined to make it sanitary, it can be sold as "turbinado" sugar. Brown sugar consists of sugar crystals coated with some molasses syrup. Most manufacturers make it by spraying syrup onto refined white sugar.

Turbinado and brown sugar might look and smell more healthful than white sugar. But the few additional nutrients they contain are so minuscule in quantity that they make no nutritional difference.

Honey is formed by an enzyme from nectar gathered by bees. Depending on where the nectar comes from, honey can differ slightly in composition and flavor. All honey is a blend of sugars, largely fructose and glucose. Like brown sugar, honey has a few nutrients; but again, they are scant. A person would have to consume four pounds of honey to get the recommended daily requirement of calcium, for example. And there is no evidence that honey is easier to digest than other sugars. When an individual eats table sugar, his body breaks the sucrose down into fructose and glucose, the two leading ingredients of honey.

Honey, raw sugar, brown sugar, and white sugar are all basically different forms of the same thing: *sugar*.

There is nothing unusual about the chemical composition of honey. It is broken down by the body in the same way as table sugar.

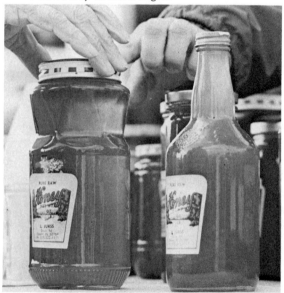

AVERAGE SUGAR CONSUMPTION

Q. *How much sugar does the average American eat?*

A. Roughly 100 pounds of sugar are consumed each year by the average American. This amount has scarcely changed in the last 50 years. Claims that sugar consumption is rising in the United States are false. Industrial sugar use has grown, but direct consumption of sugar by the consumer has declined proportionately.

According to the U.S. Department of Agriculture, sugar and other sweeteners contribute about 16.4% of our total caloric intake per year. This amounts to about 12% for adults and 20% for teenagers.

Sugar consumption at the level of 15 to 20% of total calories is considered moderate. This level, in fact, was used by the Select Committee on Generally Recognized as Safe Substances in its recommendations to the Food and Drug Administration that sugar, as currently consumed in this country, is safe.

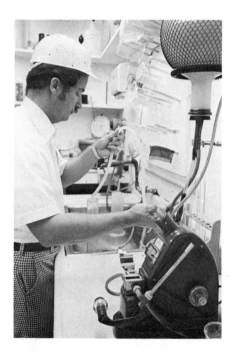

The food scientist is testing the sugar content of orange juice. Most people are not aware that eight ounces of freshly squeezed orange juice contain the equivalent of three teaspoons of sucrose.

Q. *How does the United States sugar consumption compare with that of other countries?*

A. As low-income countries experience economic growth, their rates of sugar consumption rise sharply. Evidently, as sugar becomes affordable as a source of calories, it is desired because it adds taste, variety, and attractiveness to the diet. In developing countries the demand for sugar is expected to continue to rise.

In contrast, countries with a high per capita income, such as the United States, have experienced a leveling off of sugar consumption. This indicates a natural per capita limitation to the amount of sugar consumed.

There are several countries in which sugar intake per person is higher than it is in the United States. It should be noted that some of these countries are among those with the highest life expectancy figures in the world.

Country	lbs.	Country	lbs.
New Zealand	124	United States	99
Israel	124	Sweden	96
Australia	117	Iceland	95
Denmark	108	Finland	94
United Kingdom	104	Switzerland	90
Netherlands	101	Canada	90
Ireland	100		

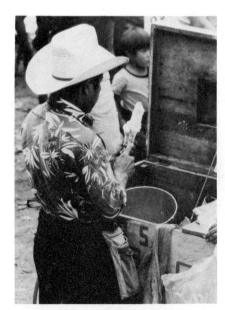

Ice cream, a favorite snack of people the world over, is dependent on sugar for many of its qualities. Sugar lowers the freezing point, which helps to keep it in a semisolid state. It contributes necessary bulk while also producing a smoother body and creamier texture.

SUGAR AND QUICK ENERGY

Q. *Should athletes eat sugar for quick energy prior to competition?*

A. It is generally a misnomer to classify a food as producing quick energy. The only time sugar would serve as quick energy for athletics would be if it were consumed after a two-day fast. The body has sizable reserves of glycogen, approximately 1,500 to 2,000 calories, which supply energy for athletic performance. If an athlete eats sugar before exercising, the sugar simply will be metabolized and moved into storage with his other fuel reserves. Furthermore, large amounts of sugar (several ounces of honey, for example) may cause extra distention in the stomach, and the evacuation mechanism may be impaired. Problems such as cramps, nausea, and diarrhea can result.

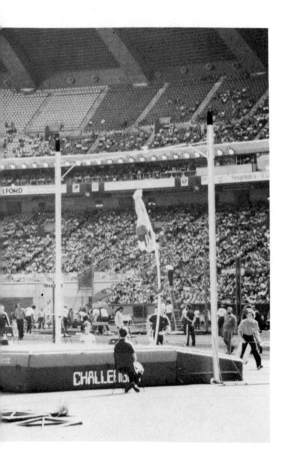

Foods produce energy. But unless a person has starved himself for several days, there are no quick-energy foods. The food that an athlete consumes on the day of competition is metabolized and stored for use several days later. (Photo by David Ponsonby)

SAFETY OF SUGAR

Q. *Do we eat too much sugar?*

A. Cautioned since childhood against eating too many sweets, many of us continue to feel guilty about consuming sugar. The irrational feeling persists that a substance so pleasant to the taste cannot possibly be good for us. It is necessary, however, to understand that sugar is but one component of a complex dietary picture involving many nutrients.

Carbohydrates provide 45 to 50% of the total calories in the American diet today. Sugar and other sweeteners account for 16.4% of our total intake, with sucrose contributing 12%. Recent surveys indicate that we are receiving more than adequate amounts of protein, too much fat, too much alcohol, and not enough carbohydrate. Carbohydrates are the only source of available calories in which an increase in consumption is indicated. If Americans were to increase consumption of total carbohydrate, and per capita sugar consumption remained constant, the percentage of total carbohydrate calories contributed by sugar would naturally decrease.

VALUE OF SUGAR

Q. *What does sugar contribute to the diet?*

A. *Sugar is a source of carbohydrates.* Sugar and starch belong to the group of nutrients called carbohydrates. Carbohydrates, together with the remaining nutrient groups—proteins, fats, vitamins, minerals, and water—make up our food and drink.

Carbohydrates are the cheapest and most easily digested form of animal and human energy. Although fat and protein can replace carbohydrate as a source of energy for most of the cells of the body, some carbohydrate is essential for humans. Carbohydrate from food is converted by the body primarily into the simple sugar, glucose. Brain, nerve, and lung tissue require glucose as their source of energy.

Nutritionists are in general agreement that 50–60% of our calories should come from carbohydrates. Sugar makes up approximately one-third of the U.S. carbohydrate intake. If one could eliminate sugar from the diet, or even cut it down, it would be difficult to find substitute sources of calories.

Sugar is a source of calories. Energy, as measured in calories, is the first need of the body. If a child gets adequate protein, but does not get sufficient calories, his body will simply burn much of that protein as fuel. The protein-sparing effect of sugar and other carbohydrates is an important consideration if the supply of protein is limited. Sugar provides an inexpensive, readily available source of calories.

Sugar makes food palatable. It is no secret that the sweet taste of sugar is almost universally pleasing. What deserves emphasis is the contribution sugar's palatability makes to overall nutrition.

Scientists are just beginning to explore the importance of taste to nutrition. Pleasant taste stimuli, including the sweet taste, have been found to affect favorably the activity of the

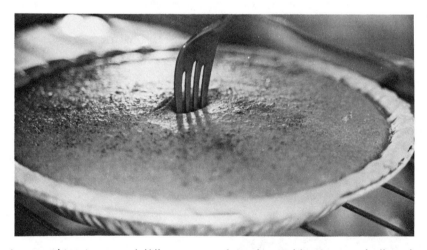

In pumpkin pie, sugar fulfills a variety of needs. It adds necessary bulk and texture and enhances the flavor of the pumpkin and spices. Sugar also contributes to crust color and flavor.

digestive system. The available evidence indicates that appealing flavor in food is particularly important to very young children. Newborn infants, in fact, exhibit a decided preference for sweetness, leading scientists to conclude that our own desire for sweets is inborn.

Obviously, no matter how nutritious a food is, it must be acceptable in order for people to eat it. Sugar can be an important factor in promoting the palatability of diets that provide a desirable distribution of calories from protein, fat, and carbohydrate. A moderate intake of sugar, then, is indispensable to good nutrition.

Sugar is an important ingredient in many processed foods. The variety of foods in which sugar is an ingredient is a reflection of the many functions it performs in addition to its sweetening effect. Sugar acts as a preservative in processed fruits, jams, and preserves. Used in small amounts, sugar has the ability to enhance the flavors in foods such as preserved meats. It is sugar that contributes necessary bulk and texture to ice cream, baked goods, and confectionery. In bread, sugar contributes to crust color and flavor and holds moisture in the product so that shelf life is extended.

It is sugar's versatility that makes it an indispensable ingredient in many of our most popular foods.

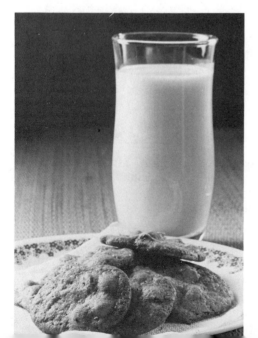

Sugar makes cookie dough easier to spread. It contributes to the taste, color, and texture of the finished product.

EMPTY CALORIES

Q. *Are calories from sugar empty calories?*

A. Since calories are a measure of heat and energy, it is technically meaningless to say they are empty. This term, however, is commonly applied to foods that contribute only calories as compared with foods that contribute other nutrients along with calories.

Refined sugar is a source of carbohydrate that has often been labeled *empty calories* because it contains no other nutrients. Fats and alcohol have also been so labeled.

Nutritionists fear that overconsumption of foods that supply calories but few nutrients dilute the diet and may result in nutritional deficiency. But fears that sugar has displaced other nutrients to the point of deficiency may be groundless. A recent study of nutrient intakes in the United States shows that our consumption of key vitamins and minerals has not decreased during this century.

Nutritionists caution us against overconsumption of calories while recommending that we combine a variety of foods to achieve a balanced intake of nutrients. Sugar can help us with this task by rendering many nutritious foods palatable. Besides, most of us consume sugar in combination with other foods and not alone.

SUGAR AND TOOTH DECAY

Q. *What effect does sugar have on the teeth?*

A. It has been stated and restated that sugars cause dental caries. The danger in accepting such statements at face value, however, is that they encourage an oversimplified view of the problem of tooth decay and its possible solutions.

Tooth decay is a complex disease. Sugar consumption is one of the many factors involved in its etiology. Other factors include heredity; the shape, alignment, and hardness of the teeth; the presence or absence of certain trace nutrients in the diet; the chemistry of the saliva; the presence of microorganisms in the mouth; and dental hygiene.

Research has shown that total sugar content of the diet is not as important as several more potent factors, such as the form of the food and the frequency with which it is consumed. Stickier foods are potentially more harmful to teeth than nonsticky foods. Frequent consumption of food between meals is more detrimental because total time of exposure is increased. There is less risk of increased caries when sugar is consumed with meals.

In view of these factors, the need for effective oral hygiene in controlling tooth-adhering plaque and bacteria becomes apparent. It is important to:

- Practice good dental hygiene, including regular visits to the dentist.
- Avoid sticky foods containing sugar between meals and at bedtime, and opt for sweets in liquid or quick-dissolving forms.
- Add fluoride to community water supplies to harden young teeth early. It is estimated that for 20–25¢ per person annually, community water supplies can be fluoridated so that 60–70% of dental decay can be eliminated.

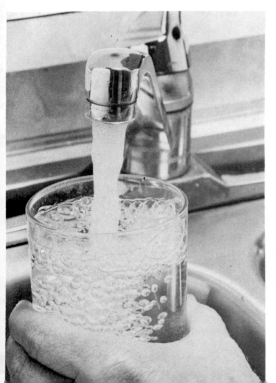

Fluoridated tap water is scientifically accepted as a safe, economical, and efficient way to prevent tooth decay.

SUGAR AND DIABETES

Q. *Is there any relationship between sugar consumption and diabetes?*

A. There has been no scientific evidence to show that sugar consumption is a specific cause of diabetes. Like all diseases, diabetes is multifactoral in origin. It would be extremely difficult to single out any one factor as its cause. Of the many factors that can increase risk of the disease, the most important seem to be obesity and genetic factors.

LOW BLOOD SUGAR

Q. *What about low blood sugar? Is it caused by consuming too much sugar?*

A. Low blood sugar is a symptom, not a disease. A person feels it when he is hungry, since it is one of the signals by which the brain learns that he needs to eat. Most people respond by having a meal or a snack.

True spontaneous low blood sugar (hypoglycemia is the medical term) is an extremely rare disease condition in which the pancreas habitually oversecretes insulin. As a result, the person's blood glucose is periodically too low. Such an individual should eat high-protein foods frequently and exclude simple sugars. Very few people are truly hypoglycemic in this sense. But all of us experience low blood sugar levels that prompt us to eat. Hunger usually is best met by consuming a balanced meal rather than a concentrated sugar snack.

SUGAR AND ADDICTION

Q. *Can individuals become addicted to sugar?*

A. Sugar addiction is a misleading phrase that has been popularized to describe individuals who overindulge in sweets. There is no scientific evidence that sugar is addictive. Recent scientific research, in fact, demonstrates that our liking for sweets is predetermined by innate factors rather than external stimuli.

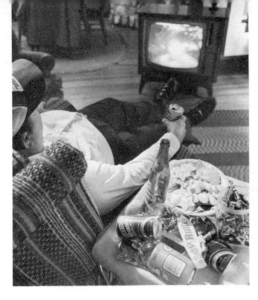

People are addicted to food, not sugar.

Scientists feel that the desire for sweets is probably the result of a basic biological drive. It is believed that this drive enables wild animals, including primitive man, to select safe foods such as fruits, while avoiding toxic substances that are bitter. Pleasure in eating is indispensable to good nutrition and sugar's sweet taste makes a significant contribution to the total diet.

SACCHARIN

Q. *What is the status of saccharin? Is it safe to use?*

A. The Food and Drug Administration currently recommends that people restrict their intake of saccharin to no more than one gram a day. This amounts to seven 12-ounce cans of diet soda or 60 small saccharin tablets a day—considerably more than anyone is probably taking.

The Food and Drug Administration has set limits on the amounts of saccharin that can be added in the manufacture of diet foods. The amount a product contains must be clearly stated on the label. Thus, a person can be aware of his daily saccharin intake.

The actions of the Food and Drug Administration followed a preliminary report that bladder tumors were discovered in animals fed the equivalent of 875 bottles of diet soda per day. If this finding is verified as significant, the government can

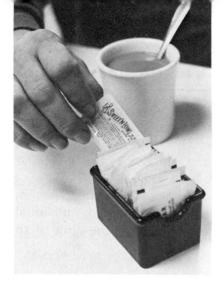

Saccharin is among the few artificial sweeteners presently allowed on the market in the United States. Molecule per molecule, saccharin is 300 times sweeter than sucrose.

invoke the so-called Delaney clause to ban saccharin despite its history of safe use by humans for the last 80 years. (For example, studies of diabetics who have used large amounts of the sweetener for up to 25 years reveal no unusual excess in cancer incidence.)

The government's recommendation of no more than one gram of saccharin a day seems an adequate guideline for fitness-minded people.

FRUCTOSE

Q. *Much is being written about fructose. What is it?*

A. Fructose is a single sugar (monosaccharide). Glucose and galactose are also in this classification. Sucrose is a double sugar (disaccharide) composed of glucose and fructose.

Fructose is the predominant sugar in honey, fruits, and vegetables. It contains exactly the same number of calories, gram for gram, that sucrose does. But fructose tastes one and a half times sweeter than sucrose.

Q. *How is fructose manufactured?*

A. Recent advances in food science have permitted the production of large amounts of fructose by the utilization of enzyme technology. Most people are familiar with corn syrup. This high-glucose sweetener is produced from cornstarch and is not considered to be very sweet tasting. By running the corn syrup over a bed of enzyme protein the glucose is converted to fructose. The resulting high-fructose corn syrup is much sweeter than glucose syrup. A similar process has been perfected with beet sugar.

Many supermarkets now offer fructose in granular, tablet, or liquid form. But before buying fructose an individual should be aware that it costs at least five times the price of an equal amount of table sugar.

FRUCTOSE VS. SUCROSE

Q. *Are there any advantages to consuming fructose instead of sucrose?*

A. Not for normal individuals. Diabetics may benefit from consuming fructose since, at low levels, it does not require insulin to be removed from the blood. What should be understood, however, is that a good percentage of the fructose is converted to glucose by the liver and intestinal lining and released into the bloodstream. Fructose, therefore, is not a panacea for treating diabetes though there are times when a physician might prescribe inclusion of fructose in the diet. In addition, fructose is being promoted as an aid for weight reduction—which it is not.

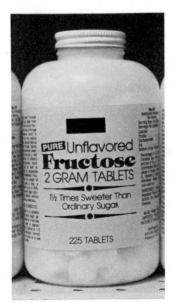

Contrary to the health food literature, fructose is not a special sweetener that is tolerated by the body better than sucrose.

FACTS ABOUT SUGAR

Q. *Can the facts about sugar be summarized?*
A. The facts about sugar's place in the diet are as follows:

- Sugar is a substance found naturally in a wide variety of plant foods. The body does not distinguish between sugar that comes from the sugar bowl and sugar that exists in fruits and vegetables.
- Sugar is a significant source of dietary carbohydrate. Carbohydrates are the body's primary energy source.
- Sugar's physical and chemical properties make it extremely useful in the preparation of a wide variety of foods by both the food industry and the household user.
- Sugar, in certain forms, contributes to the problem of dental caries. But it is only one of many factors that play a role in this disease.
- Sugar is safe. Its consumption is not related to any death-dealing disease.
- Sugar's sweet taste contributes to the pleasure of eating.

In the final analysis, sugar is neither better nor worse than any other food. It is simply one component of a balanced diet.

11

---

bread

BREAD MAKING

Q. *How is bread made?*

A. Most of the world's bread is made from such grains as rice, wheat, rye, barley, oats, and corn. In the United States, though, the preference has always been for bread made from wheat.

Originally, grain was converted to flour by grinding it between stones. This produced flour that was coarse and grayish in appearance and made unattractive bread. About 1870, stone grinding was replaced by roller mills in which steel rollers replaced stones. This change made possible finer milling in greater quantities than could be produced with stones.

Basic principles of bread making have changed little over the years. What is done today is much the same as what was done in ancient Egypt. First, flour is moistened with water to make dough. Yeast is then added prior to baking. If left at a warm temperature, the yeast ferments and causes the bread to rise. Then the bread is kneaded and put into an oven to bake where it rises once again.

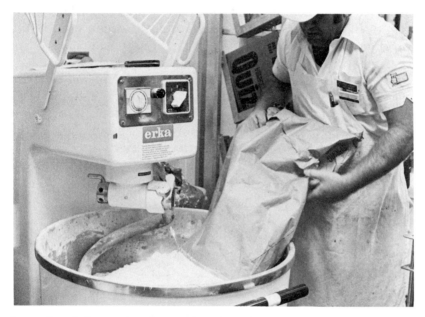

In modern bakeries dough is made in large, automated mixers by combining flour with water, yeast, and other ingredients.

After the dough is prepared, it is rolled and shaped by hand, coated with oil, and readied for baking.

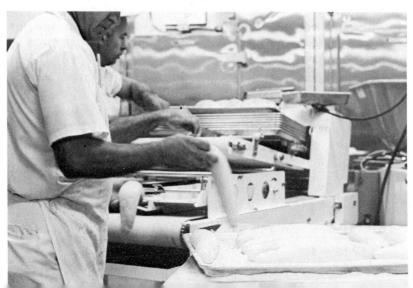

WHOLE GRAIN, ENRICHED, AND FORTIFIED

Q. *In the supermarket, the terms* whole grain, enriched, *and* fortified *can be found on the bread labels. What do the terms mean?*

A. The term *whole grain*, which can apply to wheat, rice, rye, or oats, means that the entire grain has been used in the product. *Restored* and *enriched* are interchangeable terms that mean certain nutrients lost in the processing procedure (iron and three B vitamins—riboflavin, thiamin, and niacin) have been replaced to the levels found in whole grain.

When nutrients other than these are added, or the amounts added are higher than the maximum levels established by the federal government, the term *fortified* is used.

Individuals who do a lot of home baking should use enriched or whole-grain flour whenever possible. Those who use convenience products should buy biscuit mixes, cake mixes, and refrigerated products that are made with enriched or whole-grain flour. They should do the same with packaged rolls, crackers, and cookies.

ENRICHMENT PROCESS

Q. *Why was enrichment of bread begun?*

A. In the 1920s and 1930s numerous cases of beriberi, pellagra, and riboflavin deficiency were seen in the United States. The number of Americans suffering from B complex deficiency was estimated to be one-third of the total population. There were more than 200,000 cases of pellagra in the southern United States, with beriberi and riboflavin deficiencies widespread. In 1928 there were 7,000 deaths in the United States from pellagra alone.

Reliable surveys revealed that the average American diet of the 1930s contained only one-third the amount of thiamin as when stone-ground flour was the only flour available.

As a result of these deficiencies, nutritionists started to try to convert the public to whole-wheat flour from white flour.

Much to the dismay of these determined nutritionists, people continued to find white bread and flour more attractive. The public seemed to be oblivious to nutrition.

Scientists began discussing enrichment of bread and cereal products as early as 1936. However, it was not until the Nutrition Conference for Defense, held in Washington in 1941, that the national program for the enrichment of bread and flour was officially inaugurated. The enrichment of white bread was adopted as the easiest, simplest, least expensive way of restoring certain nutrients to the diets of the greatest number of people. Of the Basic Four Food Groups, bread represented the most widely used of all foodstuffs. This was particularly true for those on limited food budgets.

Q. *How successful has the enrichment program been in eliminating certain nutritional diseases?*

A. In 1943 the death rate for pellagra was one per 100,000 population. Seven years later the death rate had dropped to 0.2 per 100,000. That year there were only 260 reported cases of pellagra. In 1960 data at the Hillman General Hospital in Birmingham, Alabama, revealed that not a single pellagrin was found in this area where pellagra was once rampant.

Similar findings were also recorded in a large general hospital in Chicago where beriberi was always a problem. A three-year search failed to reveal a single case of beriberi. In fact, twenty-five years after bread enrichment started in the United States, the serious deficiency diseases decreased to a point that it became difficult to find any cases at all.

By the latter part of the 1960s, however, the eating habits of this nation had changed considerably. As people became more affluent and transient, dietary habits were modified. Americans gradually increased their intake of meat and fat and decreased their consumption of bread and cereal. This caused flour consumption to drop from 200 pounds per person in 1910 to 100 pounds per person per year in the sixties.

The result of the reduced intake of bread and cereal was seen in the recent USDA Ten State Nutritional Study. This study revealed that some segments of our population were eating iron-rich foods and other nutrients in amounts below the RDAs.

Naturally, this opened the door to the food fad promoters. Unfortunately, these faddists are adept at mixing just enough established facts with fallacies to deceive unsuspecting persons.

Food faddists constantly claim the superiority of whole wheat bread over enriched white bread. While whole wheat bread is indeed nutritious, there is little difference between it and white bread that has been enriched. The obvious answer to the elimination of certain nutritional diseases is not the consumption of whole wheat bread rather than enriched white bread, but the eating of more bread and cereal products.

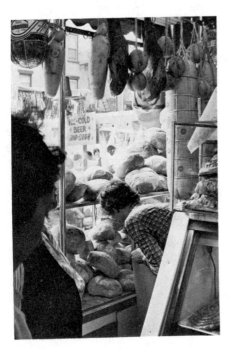

According to Dr. Mark Hegsted, chairman of the Food and Nutrition Board, Americans should eat more bread—of all kinds.

Q. *What are the major nutritional elements of enriched bread?*

A. The major elements are niacin, riboflavin, thiamin, protein, carbohydrate, and calcium. A brief description of these nutrients follows:

Niacin—helps the body utilize energy from carbohydrates and contributes to alertness.

Riboflavin—aids in growth; essential for healthy skin and eyes.

Thiamin—helps in the utilization of carbohydrates and is required to keep nerves healthy.

Iron—essential for good red blood; helps prevent anemia.

Protein—vital to good growth, strong muscles.

Carbohydrate—an ideal source of energy.

Calcium—important for strong bones, sound teeth.

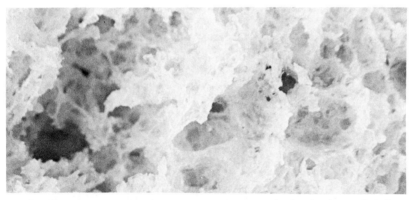

Bread is a porous food as this close-up photograph clearly shows. It is low in calories and high in nutrients.

Q. *How can bread be nutritious when milling takes out many nutrients and only four of them are replaced?*

A. It is true that levels of nutrients are decreased in milling wheat into flour. Minute amounts of sodium, magnesium, manganese, and other trace elements are lost in milling.

There are numerous food sources for these lost nutrients. Enrichment was never intended to return all the nutritional elements removed in the milling process. Enrichment was designed to correct certain nutritional deficiencies. It does that by returning the three B vitamins and iron.

With rising food prices, bread is a real bargain. Gram for gram a consumer will find bread costs considerably lower than those for hamburger, cheese, potatoes, tuna, chicken, eggs, or milk.

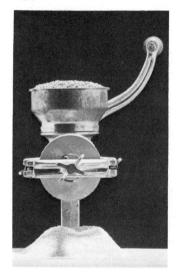

Some people prefer to make their bread at home using grain that has been converted to flour by do-it-yourself, stone-grinding mills. This can be an enjoyable experience that results in nutritious bread.

Q. *Aren't the enrichment ingredients "chemical" and "synthetic" additives?*

A. Yes, but nothing is wrong with their being "chemical" or "synthetic." Unfortunately, food faddists have promoted only the so-called "natural" and "organic" vitamins and minerals as being acceptable. This claim is unfounded. A nutrient has a certain chemical structure, regardless of whether it is synthetically produced or naturally occurring. If the structure is not identical, it is not the same substance. What most people fail to realize is that the human body is composed of chemicals, many different chemicals, all working together.

PREFERENCE FOR WHITE BREAD

Q. *Do Americans still prefer white bread over other varieties of bread?*

A. According to a survey reported in *Milling and Baking News,* white bread is still the favorite of 51% of all bread buyers in the United States. Nearly 24% of the people named whole wheat as their favorite and 10% chose rye. The remaining 15% divided their preferences among such breads as French, whole grain, raisin, bran, pumpernickel, stone-ground, and fiber.

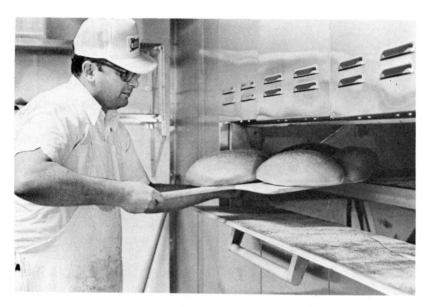

Freshly baked loaves of bread are being removed from the oven.

The survey showed that more and more people are trying and liking variety breads. White bread had been almost exclusively consumed in the 1960s. Much of the trend centers around the belief that whole wheat bread is more nutritious than white bread.

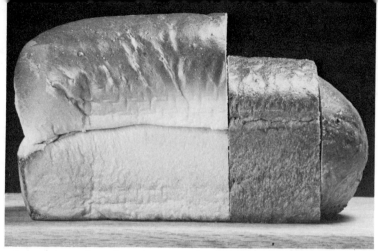

Of all bread purchased in the United States, 51% is still enriched white bread. Whole wheat is next in popularity with 24% followed by rye at 10%.

WHOLE WHEAT VS. WHITE BREAD

Q. *Is whole wheat bread superior to enriched white bread in nutritional quality?*

A. White bread has become the bread that everybody loves to knock. Critics usually describe it as a spongy, tasteless loaf that shortchanges people nutritionally. While white bread may be spongy and tasteless to some people, from a nutritional point of view there are no significant differences between whole wheat bread and enriched white bread. When cost is considered, white bread is definitely the best value for the money. Dr. Fredrick Stare of the Department of Nutrition at Harvard University reflected the opinion of most nutritionists when he stated: "I don't know of any evidence to support the idea that whole wheat products are superior nutritionally in man compared with enriched flours."

Enriched bread, when thiamin, niacin, riboflavin, and iron have been added, and when milk solids are used in baking, provides practically the same values of thiamin, niacin, and iron as whole wheat bread. It also gives twice as much riboflavin, and a great deal more calcium because of the milk that is absent from whole wheat bread.

One small problem with whole wheat bread is that it contains high levels of phytic acid. Phytic acid can bind up essential minerals—including calcium, iron, zinc, and magnesium—so that they are less available for absorption.

Even though whole wheat bread may be full of nutrients, some of the minerals it contains cannot be absorbed by the body because of the phytic acid. Even so, whole wheat bread is nutritious.

Another factor to consider is the cost of whole wheat versus white bread. A recent trip to a supermarket in Florida revealed that the typical one-pound loaf of whole wheat bread sold for 89¢, while white was 50¢. Whole wheat costs almost 80% more than an equal amount of white bread.

Where bread is concerned, a person can eat what appeals to him—white, dark, French, Italian—just as long as the label states whole-grain or enriched.

BREAD AND DIETING

Q. *Is bread a calorie-filled or "fattening" food?*

A. Actually, bread provides only a small number of calories. An average slice of enriched white bread contains about 70 calories. In a reducing diet the aim is to cut down on calories while maintaining the intake of the necessary nutrients. Bread should be a part of every reducing diet.

The real reason why the majority of people relate bread to fattening food is not the bread itself, but what they put on it. An ordinary pat of butter increases the caloric value of that slice of bread by 100 calories. Now the bread provides 170 calories, yet the actual bread contributes slightly more than one-third of the total. Add a slice of cheese to it and the caloric content goes up an additional 115. That cheese sandwich now packs a hefty 285 calories, but the caloric contribution of the bread remains at 70. Bread is not fattening; it is simply an innocent vehicle for the high-calorie foods that many people heap on top of it.

Q. *It is amazing that bread can be used on a reducing diet. How is this possible?*

A. Amazing as it may seem to some people, most nutritionists highly recommend that bread be included in a reducing

diet. An interesting study under the direction of Dr. Olaf
Mickelsen, Professor of Food Science and Human Nutrition at
Michigan State University, merits mention.

Dr. Mickelsen took two groups of eight obese college men.
For eight weeks he fed all the men 12 slices of bread daily
plus whatever else they wanted for meals and snacks. One
group lost an average of 19.4 pounds per man and the other
lost 13.7 pounds per man.

Losing weight while eating so much bread seems hard to
believe. An estimate of the total day's caloric intake may
clarify these results. At about 70 calories per slice, 12 slices
would provide about 840 calories and an estimated 30–50% of
the daily protein need. Adding another 800 calories from
meats, milk, vegetables, and fruit would total about 1,600
calories and probably furnish the balance of the daily nutrient
need. Since active young men usually require about 2,500
calories for weight maintenance, it is reasonable that body fat
should disappear at the rate of one to two pounds per week.
The success of the bread diet is probably due to its filling
bulk, which limits the amount of other foods that can be
eaten comfortably.

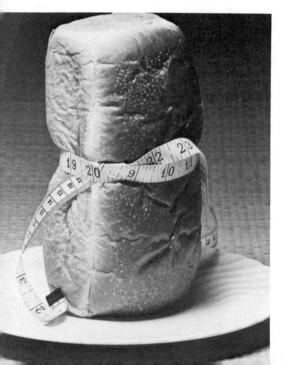

Contrary to what many weight-
conscious people believe, bread is
low in calories. Several slices of
bread daily should always be included in a reducing diet.

These results may surprise those who advocate low-carbohydrate diets for weight reduction. The calories in bread come primarily from carbohydrates. A typical slice of bread furnishes 15 grams of carbohydrate, two grams of protein, and less than one gram of fat. The men on the bread diet lost weight without any of the fatigue, hunger pangs, nausea, or headaches usually associated with low-carbohydrate diets.

RECOMMENDATIONS FOR BREAD

Q. *How much bread does a fitness-minded individual need each day?*

A. The Food and Nutrition Board recommends at least four servings a day from the bread-cereal group. One serving equals one slice of bread, or any one of the following: one-half cup of rice or pasta; five two-inch saltines; one muffin, biscuit, or small roll; two pancakes; four pieces of melba toast; three-fourths cup of unsweetened puffed or flaked dry cereal; two graham crackers; or a cup of popcorn.

Dr. Mark Hegsted, chairman of the Food and Nutrition Board, plainly states that the American people would be better off if they ate more bread. Certainly this would be advantageous to the average American who is suffering or will suffer from heart disease, since bread contains little fat and no cholesterol.

In addition, bread should be especially important to the fitness-minded individual. The starch in bread is an ideal source of energy since is it slowly broken down into glucose. Bread is of great help in the energy production process. From a health standpoint, it is and always will be the cornerstone of the Basic Four Food Groups.

12

salt

SODIUM CHLORIDE, AN ESSENTIAL NUTRIENT

Q. *What is the chemical composition of salt?*

A. Common table salt is composed of two elements, sodium and chloride. Salt is an essential part of the human diet. As it dissolves in water, it is broken into sodium and chloride ions. In all mammals the sodium ion is required to maintain the pressure and volume of the blood. It is also essential in controlling the passage of water into and out of the body's cells and the relative volumes of fluids inside and outside those cells. In addition, sodium is needed for the transmission of nerve impulses and for the metabolism of carbohydrates and proteins.

The chloride ion, too, is essential. It is involved in maintaining the acid-base balance in the blood and the passage of water across cell walls to maintain proper concentration of various chemicals. Chloride is necessary for activating certain essential enzymes, and for the formation of hydrochloric acid in the stomach, needed in the digestive process.

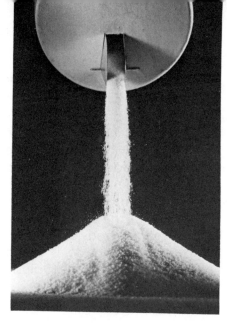

Table salt is composed of two essential minerals—sodium and chloride.

SALT REQUIREMENTS

Q. *How much salt is required in the human body each day?*
A. The exact amount of salt required by a human has been difficult to assess. The most frequent estimate of the minimum daily requirement of sodium is 200 milligrams. Since table salt is 39% sodium, this amounts to 0.5 gram of salt.

The average American daily diet almost never supplies less than the minimum requirement of salt. In fact, the total daily intake of the average American is estimated to be in the range of 10 to 12 grams of salt (3,900 to 4,700 milligrams of sodium).

The minimum daily requirement for sodium has been estimated at 200 milligrams. This is the amount found in 0.5 grams of salt, which is shown in the photograph. Most Americans get considerably more than that amount in the food they eat.

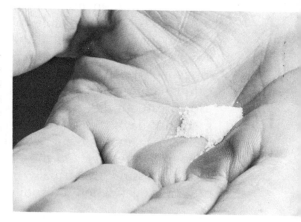

Q. *What happens to this extra salt in the body? Is it stored?*

A. Sodium and chloride are not normally stored in the body, even when the intake of salt is high. Excess amounts are excreted so that the sodium level in the body is maintained within narrow limits, as is the chloride level. The primary route of excretion is via the urine, with substantial amounts lost in the sweat and feces. About 50% of the sodium in the human body is located in the extracellular body fluids, 10% inside the cells, and 40% in the bones. Chloride is found principally in the gastric juice, blood, and other body fluids.

SALT AND HEALTH

Q. *Why has there been so much concern lately about excessive salt intake and health?*

A. Much of this concern is about dietary sodium and hypertension or high blood pressure. Hypertension afflicts more than 20% of the population of the world. It is estimated that there are 24 million cases in the United States alone. In about 90% of the cases studied, the actual cause of hypertension cannot be determined. These patients are referred to as suffering from essential or primary hypertension. Since the sodium ion plays such a major role in the physiological regulations of body fluids, it is reasonable to assume that it is capable of influencing blood pressure.

Research on the possible role of sodium in essential hypertension has been going on for some 60 years. It is not generally believed that sodium *causes* hypertension. But it has long been known that the blood pressure of many unmedicated patients with essential hypertension will lower when they are fed a diet severely restricted in sodium (below one gram per day). It is also known that their blood pressure will increase again when substantial amounts of sodium are reinstituted in the diet. On the other hand, people with normal blood pressure will usually *not* show an increase in blood pressure, even when fed sodium-rich diets.

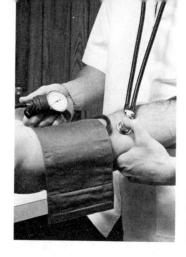

People with high blood pressure should be under a physician's care. The physician is likely to put such patients on a low-sodium diet.

DIURETICS AND SODIUM

Q. *How do diuretics influence body sodium?*

A. Hypertension is often treated with diuretics. These are substances that enhance excretion of excess sodium and water. Prolonged use of most diuretics, however, results in loss of body potassium. Thus, individuals taking diuretics are usually encouraged to eat plenty of potassium-rich foods.

BALANCING SODIUM AND POTASSIUM

Q. *Is it true that American diets are high in sodium and low in potassium?*

A. Estimates of average daily consumption of sodium and potassium indicate that sodium intake greatly exceeds that of potassium among people in developed countries. Studies with laboratory animals and observations of selected population groups strongly suggest that this is not an ideal dietary mix. A more desirable ratio could be achieved through daily consumption of much less sodium and careful attention to the selection of potassium-rich foods. Sodium is so widely distributed in foods that it is very easy to meet the body's need for sodium without adding salt.

Most people appreciate the taste of salt. Taste preference for saltiness is primarily a result of social and dietary custom and usage. Recognition of undesirably high levels of salt in infant diets has brought about a reduction in the sodium content of manufactured baby foods. Parents should avoid the needless addition of salt to the baby's food. An adult's taste preference for saltiness is often not a reliable indicator of the infant's need.

With increased use of processed and convenience foods, the individual has somewhat less control over sodium and potassium intake. During the canning and freezing of foods, sodium is often added and potassium reduced. Much of the potassium naturally present in vegetables goes into the water used in the cooking or canning process. For this reason, it is a good idea to use as little water as possible in cooking and to save leftover liquid for soups and stews.

Excessive intake of sodium should be avoided. Drastic restriction of sodium intake, however, is unwise unless recommended by a physician. Adequate dietary sodium is especially important during pregnancy. Significant sweat losses of both sodium and potassium may occur in athletes or persons doing heavy work in hot climates. An adequate intake of potassium and sodium is especially important for these individuals.

One way to prevent waste of nutrients in the kitchen is to save the liquid from canned vegetables and use it in soup stock.

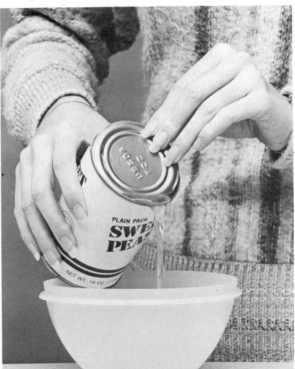

SODIUM AND POTASSIUM FOOD SOURCES

Q. *What foods are sources of sodium and potassium?*

A. Sodium occurs naturally in many foods. Common dietary sources of added sodium are sodium chloride, monosodium glutamate (MSG), soy sauce, and the common leavening agents (baking soda and baking powder). Processed products tend to be higher in sodium than fresh foods. Water supplies vary considerably in sodium content and may make a significant contribution to the total daily intake.

These foods are outstanding sources of potassium and are also very low in sodium: oranges, bananas, raisins, potatoes, and squash. Significant amounts of potassium are contributed by many other fruits, certain vegetables, milk, lean meats, poultry, fish, and whole-grain breads and cereals.

It is desirable for people with high blood pressure to strive toward a one-to-one ratio between sodium and potassium in the diet. For example, peas are high in potassium and low in sodium. Cheese is high in sodium and low in potassium.

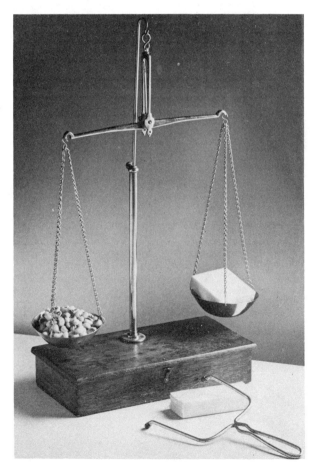

Sodium and Potassium Sources*

Meat Group		
Food	Sodium	Potassium
(100g-3½ oz.-edible portion)	(mg)	(mg)
Flat fish (flounder, sole, sanddabs)	78	342
Salmon, red		
raw	48	391
canned	522	344
Shrimp	140	220
Scallops	255	396
Oysters		
raw	73	121
frozen	380	210
Beef raw	65	355
Chicken (average figure) raw	59	285
Pork raw	70	285
Ham, light cure	1,100	340
Frankfurter	1,100	230

Fruit & Vegetable Group		
Food	Sodium	Potassium
(100g-3½ oz.-edible portion)	(mg)	(mg)
Peas, green		
raw	2	316
cooked	1	196
canned, drained solids	296	96
frozen	196	150
Beans		
mature seeds, raw	19	1,196
green, raw	7	243
canned, drained solids	236	95
Lettuce	9	264
Apple, raw	1	110
Applesauce	2	65
Banana	1	370
Orange raw	1	200
juice	1	200

Dairy Group		
Food	Sodium	Potassium
(100g-3½ oz.-edible portion)	(mg)	(mg)
Milk (cow's) whole	50	144
Buttermilk, cultured	130	140
Cheese		
cottage, creamed	229	85
uncreamed	290	72
cream	250	74
processed, American	1,136	80
Butter, salted	987	23
unsalted, less than	10	10
Margarine, salted	987	23
unsalted, less than	10	10
Eggs, whole	122	129

Bread & Cereal Group		
Food	Sodium	Potassium
(100g-3½ oz.-edible portion)	(mg)	(mg)
Wheat, raw	3	370
bran, crude	9	1,121
Shredded wheat	3	348
Flour		
whole wheat	3	370
all-purpose family	2	95
self-rising	1,079	90
Bread		
white enriched	507	85
whole wheat	527	273
Wheat flakes	1,032	
Corn flakes	1,005	120

*From The Health Letter, edited by Lawrence Lamb, Vol. X, No. 12, December 23, 1977, p. 4.

ALTERNATIVE SEASONINGS TO SALT

Q. *What are some alternative seasonings?*

A. Many pleasures await the person who is willing to experiment with the many possibilities of flavoring with spices. Preferences can also be developed for the special taste of fresh as opposed to highly processed foods. Here are a few alternatives to added salt: sweet butter and lemon juice on asparagus; green peppers, tomatoes, and chili powder with corn; dill, thyme, marjoram, nutmeg, or unsalted French dressing with green beans; onion, mushrooms, or mint with fresh peas; mace, onion, parsley, chives, or scallions with potatoes; ginger, cloves, or nutmeg with winter squash; onion and green peppers with summer squash; basil, chervil, or tarragon with tomatoes; sweet butter and dill with salmon or other fish; mushrooms and tarragon with eggs; bay leaf, cumin, or oregano with veal; rosemary with lamb; garlic and sage with pork; bay leaf, thyme, marjoram, onion, dry mustard, or nutmeg with beef; paprika or sage with chicken; fruits with almost any meat or poultry as an accompaniment or glaze.

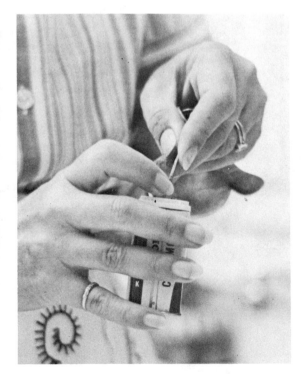

Spices can be substituted for salt in many recipes.

SALT AND FOOD PRODUCTION

Q. *What is it about salt that makes it so useful in food production?*

A. Salt serves a number of functions in food technology. It has served widely as a preservative for centuries and is essential in processing meats and cheese products. The use of salt controls certain microbial actions. For example, it allows sauerkraut to emerge from shredded cabbage or specific kinds of cheeses to form from initially identical dairy cultures. Salt controls textures and moisture levels in various foods, in addition to its obvious flavoring function.

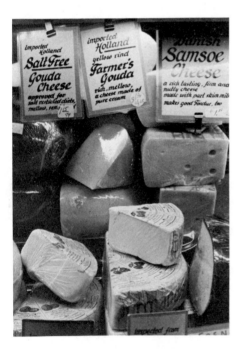

Salt is required in the processing of most cheeses.

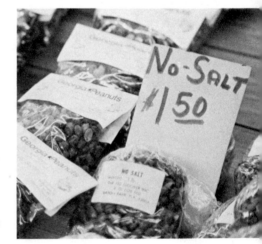

Peanuts without salt would be bland eating for most people.

DANGERS OF SALT TABLETS

Q. *Should athletes consume salt tablets during hot weather training?*

A. No, athletes should not take salt tablets. But they should certainly keep their bodies well hydrated by consuming large amounts of water before, during, and after training. If an athlete takes salt tablets when his body has too little salt, it will help retain water. If he consumes salt tablets when his body has normal amounts or too much salt, however, it will cause him to lose an increased amount of water as well as potassium.

An overdose of salt under hot, humid conditions can be more harmful than a lack of it. Too much salt in the blood can cause the most critical form of heat exhaustion. Excess salt thickens the blood, making it more likely to clot.

Normally, an athlete's taste buds protect him from consuming too much salt. But salt tablets bypass the taste-bud mechanism and a person does not know when to stop taking them. Furthermore, salt tablets may irritate the stomach lining or be passed completely undissolved.

FOOD ADDITIVES

Q. *Recently, the popular press has made people aware of the use of food additives such as monosodium glutamate and calcium propionate. Why are so many additives used in foods? Is it possible that such additives can be detrimental to athletic performance?*

A. Chemical food additives are necessary to preserve the high quality of many foods now available in the supermarket. These chemicals are added by food processors to improve or maintain quality or to give some added advantage not found in the food's fresh state but desired by the consumer.

Most consumers are unaware of the vast preparation that goes into many of the foods that are found in today's market. The time involved and distances involved in getting products from farm to manufacturers and then to consumers are some-times great. It therefore becomes difficult to keep food items at the peak of freshness throughout this entire journey unless food additives are used. Most of the additives can be grouped under the heading of nutrient supplements, flavoring agents, preservatives, emulsifiers, and stabilizers and thickeners.

The Food Additives Amendment, passed by the federal government in 1958, requires that additives be proven safe for consumption. In this respect, a variety of carefully controlled tests are made before additives can be marketed. The athlete need not be worried about certain food additives affecting performance. These additives are used in such very small amounts that one would have to consume abnormally large amounts of certain foods in order for dangers to be even remotely possible. Most of the additives are completely harm-less when consumed in normal amounts.

fast foods

POPULARITY OF FAST FOODS

Q. *How popular are fast foods?*

A. Of the 50 million Americans who eat out daily, more than a quarter choose fast food. In 1979, statistics revealed that the average adult eats in a fast-food restaurant nine times a month.

Fast food has become a lucrative business. There are more than 300 chains, comprising 60,000 outlets. The business is dominated by companies such as McDonald's, Burger King, Kentucky Fried Chicken, Wendy's, Hardee's, Tastee Freeze, Dairy Queen, and Pizza Hut. The fast-food industry amassed $20 billion in sales in 1978, about a quarter of what Americans spent to feed themselves away from home.

Although the popularity of fast foods is increasing, so is the criticism. Critics generalize by stating that fast food is notoriously high in sugar, fat, calories, and salt while low in fiber. Furthermore, they claim it is detrimental to our national well-being. What the critics do not point out is that fast food refers to a generic category of food prepared and served in rapid order. The term *fast* refers to service rather than food.

The ultimate fast food from the service point of view is human milk. When the infant cries the mother will nurse. Human milk is high in calories, fat, and sugar and low in fiber. But no one criticizes it as being hazardous to the infant's health.

RATIONALE BEHIND FAST FOODS

Q. *Why do Americans like fast foods?*

A. The popularity of fast-food restaurants seems to be tied to the American society's preoccupation with *speed* and *security*.

The speed at which food is ordered and served has become increasingly important to the busy worker. At noon workers from the factory or office begin an efficient trek to the burger shop. The ordering is easy. The cost is predictable. And in two minutes they are tucked safely into a table or car where a burger, fries, and shake can be wolfed down. The efficient worker can be back in the office in 30 minutes, or at most one hour.

Security in eating for the average American means there are no surprises. The vast majority of the fast-food outlets offer security because the customer knows his order today will have the same shape and taste that it had the week

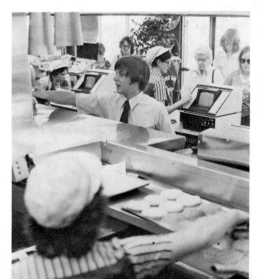

The American attachment to fast food represents a yearning for something dependable. Burgers coming off an assembly line are standardized and do not pretend to be anything more than they are.

before. Fast food is a repeat-customer business. People return time after time to order identical-tasting food in identical-sized portions. Evidently, the fast-food customer values security as much as food.

CALORIE COUNTING

Q. *How many calories are in typical fast-food meals?*

A. The average fast-food meal (burger, fries, and shake) provides about half the calories needed for an entire day by adult men, and more than half the calories required by women and children. If such a fast-food meal were added to two meals per day at other restaurants, the total caloric count would add fat to the average customer.

Calorie counts of items from popular fast-food restaurants are listed below:

McDonald's

Hamburger	251
Quarter pounder	416
Quarter pounder/cheese	523
Big Mac	561
French Fries	215
Chocolate shake	315
Fish fillet	407
Hot Apple Pie	269
Cheeseburger	310

Burger King

Hamburger	230
Whopper	630
Whopper Jr.	285
French Fries	220
Chocolate shake	365
Double Hamburger	325

Pizza Hut

Cheeze pizza	
½ 13-inch thick crust	900
½ 13-inch thin crust	850
½ 15-inch thick crust	1200
½ 15-inch thin crust	1150

NUTRIENTS IN FAST FOODS

Q. *Besides calories, how nutritious are fast-food meals?*

A. Dr. Judith Stern and R. V. Denenberg evaluated fast-food meals according to the U.S. Recommended Daily Allowances for vitamins and minerals. The following four meals are representative:

1. Super burger, regular order of french fries, vanilla shake.
2. Fried chicken (three pieces), roll, cole slaw, potatoes.
3. Half of a 10-inch pizza, iced tea with two teaspoons of sugar.
4. Fried fish sandwich, regular order of french fries, vanilla shake.

The four fast-food meals are a good source of vitamin B_1 (thiamin), B_2 (riboflavin), B_{12}, and niacin. If fortified milk products are consumed, the meals would also be adequate for children's needs for vitamin D. Adults usually get all they need from sunshine. The meals tend to be low in vitamins A, B_6, folacin (folic acid), pantothenic acid, and C. But with appropriate food choices for the rest of the day, the proper levels can be reached. For example, the individual should consume green and yellow vegetables in his other meals. Or, if the fast-food chain has a salad bar, he could add to his nutrition by selecting carrots, tomatoes, and lettuce.

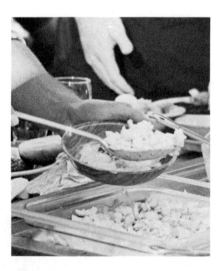

Many fast-food restaurants now offer salad bars. Vegetables and fruits help provide nutritional balance to fast-food meals.

Fast foods have ample supplies of the minerals calcium, phosphorus, sodium, iodine, and zinc. Pizza is especially high in calcium because of the cheese. Most fast foods, however, lack concentrations of the following minerals: copper, iron, magnesium, and manganese. To supply these missing nutrients, a fast-food eater would be wise to consume at other meals green leafy vegetables, fruits, nuts, and occasionally liver.

PROTEIN CONTENT

Q. *What about the protein content of fast foods?*

A. Fast-food meals are rich in protein. The average fast-food meal, for example, contains about 25 grams of protein. This amounts to 46% of a man's and 56% of a woman's daily needs. Pizza, with cheese and meat, is especially high in protein.

FAVORITE FOODS OF TEENAGERS

Q. *What are the favorite foods of teenagers?*

A. A 1979 Gallup Youth Survey found that Italian food was the overwhelming favorite of teenagers. Thirty-seven percent listed pizza as their top choice. Steak, at 30%, was next and it was followed by hamburgers, Mexican food, and french fries.

Pizza Hut has a heat-retaining carry-out carton that enables people to enjoy warm pizza at home. Two slices of a large pizza with everything on it contain approximately 500 calories.

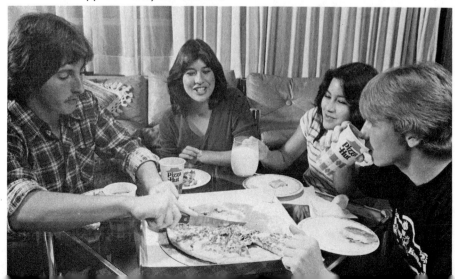

Conversely, Gallup found the least liked foods of teenagers to be, in descending order, spinach, liver, broccoli, beans, and vegetables in general.

FAST-FOOD BEVERAGES

Q. *Are the beverages sold at fast-food places nutritious?*

A. Shakes and cola drinks are the rule at fast-food restaurants. Both contain an abundance of calories. Shakes that are made with milk or an appreciable amount of fat-free milk solids would add protein and calcium to the meal. The only nutrients in cola drinks are water and carbohydrates. Most overfat people would be wise to skip the shakes and colas and drink water instead.

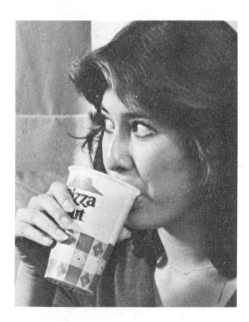

Most fast-food establishments offer a wide array of beverages, such as soft drinks, shakes, coffee, tea, milk, and orange juice.

HOT DOGS

Q. *How nutritious is a hot dog?*

A. Franks, weiners, or hot dogs are processed under rigid

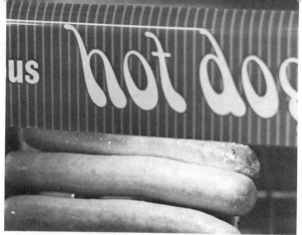

A recent food survey found that hot dogs are served in 95% of all homes in the United States. Furthermore, adults eat more hot dogs than children, and women eat more than men.

federal, state, and county inspection programs. In accordance with new USDA regulations, all hot dog ingredients must be listed on the label in decreasing order of quantity. And all formulas and package labels must be approved by federal inspectors before any hot dog may be produced.

Hot dogs are nutritionally sound. An average hot dog contains five to seven grams of protein—about the same as in one egg, but with about one-tenth the amount of cholesterol. Hot dogs also contain carbohydrates, vitamins, and trace minerals. Even when a filler such as nonfat dry milk, cereal, or soy protein is added to the meat, the nutrition is improved and the cost is less.

POTATO CHIPS

Q. *Are potato chips junk food?*

A. There are no true junk foods. Any food can be labeled as junk if it is excessively consumed. That same food, if consumed in moderation with a variety of other foods, can contribute significantly to nutritional well-being.

Potato chips are thin slices of potatoes that are fried in oil. The frying adds many calories to a nutritious, relatively low-calorie vegetable. Potato chips might be best called auxiliary foods—foods that, while not at the core of the diet, do offer some contribution to nutrition.

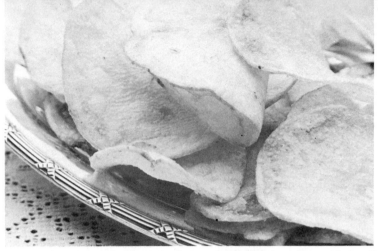

Even though potato chips are high in calories, they are nutritious. One ounce of chips contains 163 calories but includes 10% of the recommended dietary allowance for vitamin C and substantial, though lesser amounts of niacin, vitamin B$_6$, phosphorus, and magnesium.

FAST FOOD IN VENDING MACHINES

Q. *Is food obtained from vending machines always safe to eat?*

A. In recent years, there has been a phenomenal growth in the food vending industry. It is now possible to get a complete meal. At one time, the only food items associated with the vending machines were gum, candy, and similar nonperishable items. But now, vending machines distribute potentially hazardous foods. For example, milk, eggs, and meat are capable of supporting rapid growth of infectious or toxin-producing microorganisms. Not only must these foods be prepared under sanitary conditions, but they must be transported in refrigerated vehicles and dispensed in refrigerated vending machines. The foods must be replaced frequently in the vending machines and discarded should a power failure occur. A machine with slow turnover in an out-of-the-way location may contain food that is spoiled, especially if its wrapper has been broken.

Generally speaking, the food-vending industry has made great strides in ensuring that its new products are fit to eat, but problems do occur occasionally. Regulations for the sale of such foods were prepared through cooperative efforts of the National Automatic Merchandising Association, the U.S. Public Health Service, and state and local health agencies.

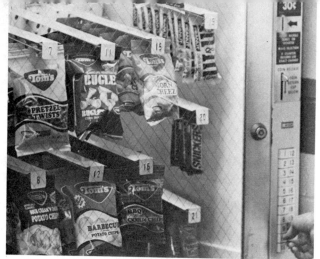

Most vending machines offer dependable, safe food.

FAST FOODS AND OBESITY

Q. *Do fast foods contribute to obesity?*

A. Obesity is the most common nutritional disorder in the United States. Obesity is caused by many factors such as genetics, lack of proper exercise, environment, socialization, and too many food calories. If an individual's daily caloric intake exceeds his caloric output, and if fast foods have been a part of his meals, then fast foods have contributed to the storage of fat within his body. The same parallel, however, can be made to any food in his diet that contained calories.

FAST FOODS AND FAT

Q. *Is it true that fast foods contain too much fat?*

A. The most popular fast food meal (a hamburger, french fries, and a shake from McDonald's) contains 59% carbohydrate, 28% fat, and 13% protein. This meal is not too high in fat. In fact, it seems perfectly designed according to the optimum diet for health described in Chapter 1.

Some fast foods, however, are high in fat. A typical fried chicken dinner or a fish sandwich and fries each provide about 50% of their calories in the form of fat. Thus, an individual who consumes certain fast food meals would need to emphasize fat-free foods such as fruits, vegetables, and grains in his other daily meals.

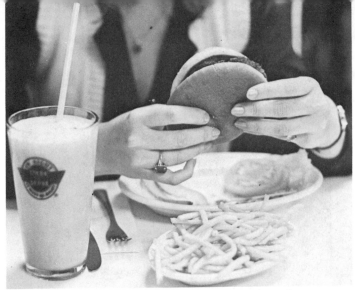

A hamburger with lettuce, tomato, pickle, onion, fried potatoes, and a vanilla milk shake is a well-balanced meal.

FAST FOOD AND GAS

Q. *Do fast foods cause gas?*

A. Internal gas or flatus is usually a result of two factors. One is swallowed air. The other is the action of bacteria in the large intestine upon certain nondigestible carbohydrates contained in foods.

Extremely gas-inducing foods include milk, onions, celery, carrots, bananas, raisins, prunes, apricots, bagels, and beans. Among moderately gas-producing foods are pastries, potatoes, eggplant, citrus fruits, apples, and bread. With the exception of some Mexican foods, fast foods are less gas-inducing than most other foods.

HAMBURGER VS. STEAK

Q. *Recently a newspaper article reported that a food scientist had claimed a hamburger, french fries, and a milk shake were equivalent to a small steak, a baked potato, and a salad. Is this correct?*

A. Yes, this statement is basically correct. Dr. Howard Appledorf, Food Science Professor at the University of Florida, has studied the nutritional aspects of fast foods in his laboratory for the last 10 years.

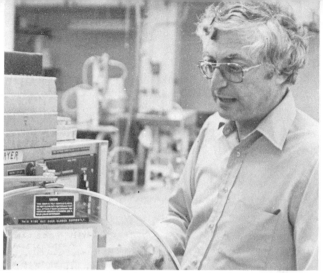
Using a freeze-drying process that converts food to a white powder for chemical analysis, Dr. Howard Appledorf has found most foods sold in fast-food establishments to be highly nutritious.

In 1969 Dr. Appledorf started a course called "Man's Food." Sixteen students signed up. Today, that class has 700 students each quarter, making it among the most popular classes at the Gainesville university campus.

Dr. Appledorf's students are often surprised when he tells them that a hamburger dinner at a fast-food restaurant is nutritionally about the same as a small New York strip steak, a baked potato, and a salad.

"No one should really be surprised at that," he insists. "A hamburger dinner is really meat, bread, and potatoes, only in different form than a steak dinner."

He admits that a hamburger dinner is somewhat low in vitamin A. "But if a kid uses ketchup on his french fries, he has sufficient vitamin A," he adds.

FAST FOODS AND ADDITIVES

Q. *Fast foods are reported to be loaded with chemicals and additives. Are these chemicals and additives detrimental to health?*

A. It is true that the foods served at chain outlets are laden with chemical additives.

Chemical additives with polysyllabic names serve a worthy purpose. They make the food taste better, look better, last longer, or stay free from germs and spoilage. More than 2,800 additives are approved for use by the federal government. It should be pointed out that, as a result of additives and other factors, the American diet is becoming safer all the time.

Data compiled by the American Cancer Society and the National Cancer Institute suggest that our eating habits are less likely to cause cancer than they once were. Deaths from stomach cancer have declined. Some of this decline can be attributed to improvements in medical care, but stomach cancer is still fatal in about 90 cases out of 100, so the decline may well be related to diet. And since the liver is the primary organ responsible for detoxifying the substances we eat, the substantial decline in liver cancer may also be due to a healthier diet that contains numerous additives.

Q. *How many pounds of additives does an average individual consume each year?*

A. The per capita consumption of food additives per year in the United States is about 136 pounds. The most widely used additive is sucrose or table sugar. Each person consumes an average of 99 pounds of sugar per year. The second most widely used additive is salt, of which we use about 15 pounds per year. After salt comes corn syrup, about eight pounds, and dextrose, four pounds. It should be noted that the 136 pounds has dwindled to 10 pounds if sugar, salt, corn syrup, and dextrose are excluded from the list. Following these are 33 different additives that account for 9 pounds a year. Of these 33, 18 are used either as leavening agents or to adjust the acidity of food. Yeast, sodium bicarbonate, citric acid, black pepper, mustard, and monosodium glutamate are among the most often used of these 16.

Our list is now down to one pound, which is spread over 1,000 or more other additives we use. The median level of use of these is about one-half a milligram per additive per year— the weight of one grain of salt per year.

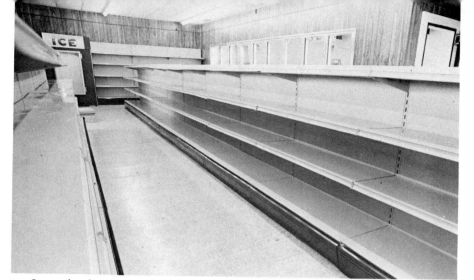

Some food scientists fear that if all additives were removed from foods, grocery stores would become almost barren within several months. The development of food additives and preservation techniques over the last few decades has been primarily responsible for our abundant food supply.

Q. *What would happen if all additives were removed from foods?*

A. Additives in foods serve a multitude of functions such as taste, looks, preservation, and protection. They also save consumers money. If additives were removed from white bread, for example, we would have to change our whole bread distribution system. This would not only waste much needed food; it would also cost the American consumer $1.1 billion per year. The removal of additives from margarine would cost $600 million. The removal of nitrates and nitrites from processed meats would cost another $600 million, and the removal of potassium sorbate from processed cheese would cost $32 million. The four products, without additives, would cost the consumer more than $2 billion per year—a sizable figure.

NITRATE-NITRITE CONTROVERSY

Q. *What is the controversy about nitrates and nitrites?*

A. Hot dogs, bacon, ham, and other packaged meats owe their appetizing color and characteristic taste largely to the

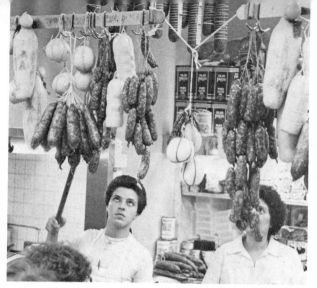

While some people complain loudly about the sodium nitrate in cured meats, they do not realize that it is found naturally in vegetables such as celery, lettuce, and radishes.

addition of nitrates and nitrites. These chemicals also inhibit the growth of the deadly bacteria known as clostridium botulinum, the cause of botulism. As a result, the refrigerator life of meats is prolonged. The nitrate-nitrite additives also make the spores of the bacteria heat-sensitive. Thus, bacteria can be killed when the meat is cooked at reasonable temperatures during processing.

Despite this contribution to public health, the nitrate-nitrite duo has fallen under suspicion. In some circumstances they can combine with substances to form another group of chemicals called nitrosamines. Nitrosamines have proved carcinogenic in laboratory animals.

Those who propose eliminating nitrates and nitrites from meat processing have run into opposition. Not only the meat packers but a number of food scientists point out that while the danger to humans from nitrosamines is still theoretical, the risk of death from botulism is quite real.

The government's regulatory policy is to control carefully the maximum levels of nitrates and nitrites that can be added to food. For example, it has banned the addition of nitrates to bacon and lowered the permissible levels of nitrites. With the addition of vitamin C to bacon, the formation of nitrosamines during cooking is inhibited.

14

health foods

HEALTH FOODS DEFINED

Q. *What are health foods?*

A. Health foods are usually thought of as being specially produced and packaged foods or supplements that are available in health food stores. Recently, the Federal Trade Commission even considered banning the term *health food* in advertising because it may fool consumers into thinking particular foods will provide good health.

Good health, with its promise of vim and vigor, is a desirable state. But the term *health* is often confused with *food*. To say that health is directly related to food is a misconception. Health is a result of many factors, just one of which is food.

The body does not require any particular food. It uses some 50 nutrients in varying amounts. No nutrient is considered a health nutrient. But any nutrient that is required for human nutrition is essential to life and health, even though some are needed in very small amounts.

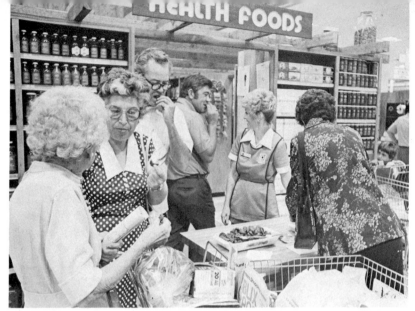

Health foods usually cost from 30 to 500% more than ordinary foods.

HISTORY OF HEALTH FOODS

Q. *How did health foods evolve?*

A. Health foods are as old as mankind. Primitive people frequently believed that a person became like what he ate. They refused to eat the flesh of a timid deer or the insidious snake and sought the hearts of lions or other brave animals. Writings before the time of Christ record how Romans thought cabbage was a miracle food.

Medicine and nutrition progressed little beyond this stage until the sixteenth century. During the sixteenth century many doctors began dissections and chemical trials on humans, which led to the formation of an alchemistic sort of secret to health. Since there was little understanding of human physiology and no sound theory of the origins of disease, the chief method of healing was to feed the patient something unusual or repulsive. Examples of unusual recommendations were worms for lung disease, deer fat for nerves, and goose fat for piles.

Settlers of the New World and later immigrants brought along their ideas on medication. Sometimes notions sprang from a panicky need to discover the reason why. In 1832 when cholera broke out on the eastern seaboard, many cities, among them New York, promptly banned the sale of fruit as fresh fruit was associated with the epidemic. Needless to say, the cholera epidemic continued.

Shortly thereafter, an ordained minister by the name of Sylvester Graham began to lecture on the benefits of vegetables and the evils of meat. He particularly advocated putting the bran back into wheat flour. Graham's ideas spread rapidly as evidenced by the popularity of the now famous graham cracker.

The twentieth century ushered in the health and breakfast cereal ideas of John H. Kellogg and Charles W. Post of Battle Creek, Michigan. Although Kellogg and Post were friends at first, they became bitter competitors and formed separate companies that manufactured cure-alls for many ailments. Many of their cereals, such as Kellogg's Corn Flakes and Post's Grape Nuts, are popular today, even though their claims are certainly less extravagant.

With the discovery of various nutrients, particularly the much publicized vitamins, a wave of cures and miracle health foods burst onto the scene. Health food stores began to spring up in the 1950s, first in California, then gradually in the large metropolitan areas of Florida, New York, Texas, and elsewhere. Throughout the 1960s, this industry grew steadily and undramatically. In 1970 *The Wall Street Journal* stated that there were 2,000 health food stores in the United States.

The health food business began to change during the 1970s. When large, well-planned malls became the shopping meccas of middle-class Americans, several chains of franchised health food stores, such as General Nutrition Centers, began to operate places of business in many of them. By 1979, there were more than 6,000 health food stores in the United States.

ORGANIC FOODS

Q. *What are organically grown fruits and vegetables?*

A. *Organically grown* is a term now applied to foods raised without manufactured fertilizers or pesticides. While such

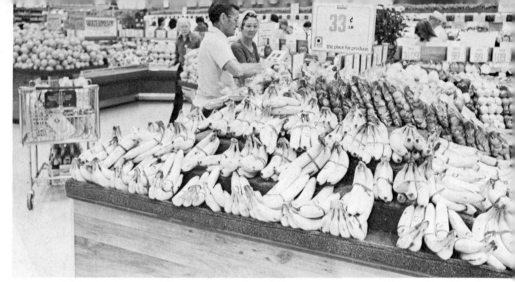

Fruits and vegetables are considered by some nutritionists to be the original health foods. Certainly, most people would profit by consuming more fruits and vegetables.

foods often cost more than the commercially grown (supermarket) fruits and vegetables, their nutrition value or nutrient content is not superior.

Actually, there is no way of being certain that foods sold or promoted as organically grown were in fact grown under those conditions. Frequently, they were not because there are not that many growers who refuse to use scientific know-how in their operations. The U.S. Department of Agriculture has been unable to find significant differences between the nutritional content of organically grown and ordinary fruits and vegetables.

Recently, Dr. Hilda White of Northwestern University noted that, if modern agricultural technology were to be discarded in favor of organic farming, the worldwide problems of hunger, malnutrition, and famine would be multiplied immeasurably.

Without chemical fertilizers, farmers would have to use twice as much land to produce the same amount of crops. Former Secretary of Agriculture Earl Butz has said 50 million people would starve to death if we went back to organic fertilizers entirely. It has been estimated that 80% of the foods in our supermarkets would become unavailable if all pesticides, herbicides, chemical fertilizers, and additives were banned.

Synthetic fertilizers and processed foods have tremendous potential for helping meet the food needs of our rapidly expanding population, but both must be used with discretion. Nutrition awareness is an excellent motivator, but it can produce fear, distrust, and a profit bonanza for some; or it can help improve health and vitality and provide a fair gain for honest businessmen. It all depends on whether people can be taught to apply basic concepts of food and nutrition.

NATURAL VS. SYNTHETIC

Q. *Is it true that rose hips provide a more nutritious source of vitamin C than synthetic vitamin C tablets?*

A. Faddists are quick to promote the vitamins from natural sources as opposed to vitamins that are produced synthetically. Nutritional research shows, however, that there are no differences between natural and synthetic vitamins, except for the higher cost of the former.

Actually, all foods are mixtures of chemicals. Chemicals are not dangerous or unnatural in themselves. The vitamin C in tablet form is identical to the naturally occurring product. Once the chemical identity of a food or nutrient is known, synthesized, and sold, many people are taught to distrust it.

Just as every food or nutrient can produce undesirable side effects if consumed in excessive quantities, so can chemicals be used unwisely. Foods or nutrients are just like drugs: They can contribute to health but they can also be abused.

WHEAT GERM

Q. *Would it be beneficial for a fitness-minded person to consume wheat germ daily?*

A. Wheat germ is the most nutritious part of the wheat plant and is often destroyed during the milling of wheat flour. It is a rich source of B vitamins, protein, and vitamin E. Many people enjoy its flavor. For example, when toasted, wheat germ becomes a tasty cereal with a nutlike flavor, or the oil can be used on salads. Some athletes even drink the oil straight from the bottle.

Claims are made that wheat germ can prevent aging, muscular dystrophy, and heart disease. Many athletes also believe that wheat germ oil increases their strength and endurance. But none of these claims that wheat germ is a unique supplier of some essential or therapeutic ingredients has been substantiated by well-controlled studies.

Again the answer is to eat a well-balanced or mixed diet. Wheat germ is not an essential food; it is not unique or magic. Enriched flour, fruits, vegetables, meat, and dairy products as well as many other foods supply the same nutrients found in wheat germ.

VITAMIN E

Q. *Vitamin E is a popular supplement sold in health food stores. Are any of the widely believed claims about vitamin E valid?*

A. Vitamin E has been claimed to grow hair on bald heads, prevent ulcers, revive sexual feelings, ease arthritis pain, and cure a host of other physical problems. Although vitamin E is an essential nutrient, there is no scientific evidence that it will do any of the dramatic things that are being claimed. Vitamin E supplements are not needed for the treatment of disease.

Vitamin E is a common household word. The interest in it is based on many unjustifiable claims being made in the popular press and health food literature—especially the unproved claim that it will increase a person's sexual potency.

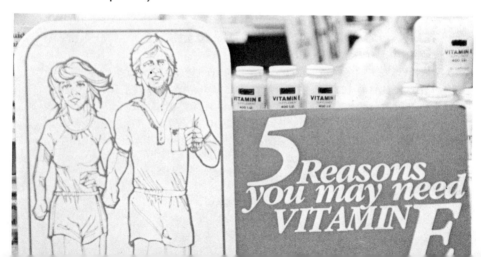

The lack of evidence that vitamin E supplements are needed by adults does not mean that nobody has investigated this in the past. Forty years ago investigators found that depriving animals of vitamin E had serious effects that varied from species to species: muscular dystrophy in chicks, rabbits, and guinea pigs; liver degeneration, growth retardation, and reproductive failure in rats; and heart damage in calves.

But deprivation of vitamin E has never produced these effects or any identifiable ailments in humans. More important, in humans already suffering from such disorders, treatment with massive amounts of vitamin E has not been shown to have a beneficial effect.

Q. *What about the cosmetic usefulness of vitamin E?*

A. In this area the claims have reached new heights. Cosmetics containing vitamin E have been promoted for healing skin blemishes, for softening dry skin, for erasing wrinkles, for giving new life to aging skin, and even for combating underarm odor. There is no evidence from controlled studies to substantiate such benefits.

Vitamin E has not been proved scientifically to have any of the miraculous effects being claimed for it. The Food and Drug Administration sees no reason for individuals in good health who eat a balanced diet to use vitamin E supplements.

FERTILE EGGS VS. REGULAR EGGS

Q. *What are fertile eggs? Are they more nutritious than regular eggs?*

A. Fertile eggs, which are supposedly available only at health food stores, are promoted as being very special and having greater nutrient content than infertile or sterile eggs. The implication of the description of fertile eggs is that there are infertile eggs being laid by sterile chickens, namely those raised in egg-laying batteries (cages). The claim is that the chicken who is unconfined and allowed to roam about, eating insects and scratching in the dirt, is able to lay a better

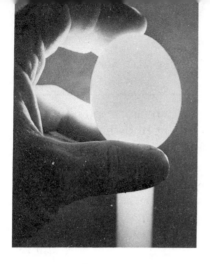

The nutritional qualities of a so-called fertile egg are exactly the same as the nutritional qualities of a regular egg. Furthermore, the color of the shell has no bearing on the nutrients of the egg.

egg. The egg-laying capacity of the hen that roams about the farmer's yard is supposed to be superior to the egg-laying capacity of the hen whose diet has been scientifically designed and carefully regulated to be sure she is receiving all the nutrients she needs.

Actually, the so-called fertile eggs should be called yard eggs—which may or may not be fertile. A person cannot be sure that eggs sold in health food stores are fertile. In order to be sure that an egg was fertile, he would have had to allow the hen to mate with a sexually potent rooster, incubate the newly laid egg for 36 hours, and then examine it under a high-power microscope to determine whether embryonic formation had begun. The truth of the matter is that both fertile and nonfertile eggs have the same nutrients, content of cholesterol and lecithin, poaching characteristics, or whatever. Of course, an individual can pay 40¢ more per dozen for fertile eggs and perhaps this will make them taste 40¢ better.

RAW MILK VS. REGULAR MILK

Q. *Is certified raw milk better than regular milk?*

A. Although certified raw milk may contain somewhat larger amounts of certain nutrients than regular homogenized and pasteurized milk, it is more expensive and dangerous to consume. Health food devotees point out that pasteurization destroys most of the beneficial hormones, enzymes, steroids, and a large portion of the fat- and water-soluble vitamins in milk. But the body is not able to absorb the large enzymes or most of the hormone molecules. Rather, it digests them to smaller molecules, absorbs them, and then synthesizes what compounds it needs. Although pasteurization destroys some nutrients in milk, it also kills dangerous bacteria. That is the whole point of pasteurization. Safe marketing of unpasteurized milk, which is free of dangerous bacteria, would require impeccable hygiene and constant supervision of cows, equipment, and employees. The greater ease of processing pasteurized milk, as well as its safer consumption, far outweighs the advantage of supplying a few more nutrients. These lost nutrients can easily be obtained in other foods.

BREWER'S YEAST

Q. *What is brewer's yeast? Is it a desirable constituent of an athlete's diet?*

A. Brewer's yeast is a bitter yellow powder that is related to a variety of yeast that is a by-product of beer brewing. It does contain large amounts of B vitamins, amino acids, and minerals. Supplementing the diet with dried brewer's yeast might be useful if an athlete is deficient in protein and B vitamins; but eating bitter yeast is not the most efficient or the most appetizing way to obtain these nutrients.

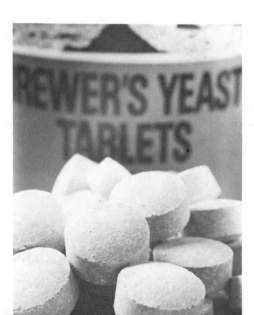

Brewer's yeast is a nutritious dietary supplement, but it has no particular virtue. A diet with a sufficient variety of food is going to be balanced without supplements.

BLACK STRAP MOLASSES

Q. *Is black strap molasses a cure for many ailments?*

A. Black strap molasses is the thick syrupy residue that is left after sugar cane has been refined into white sugar. Unlike honey and table sugar, which provide only empty calories, black strap molasses does contain calcium, iron, and most of the B vitamins. But claims that black strap molasses can prevent cancer and cure ulcers, varicose veins, arthritis, and any other trouble have not been authenticated and should be ignored.

YOGURT

Q. *Will yogurt help a person digest food more completely?*

A. Yogurt is a fermented milk product. Like all dairy products, it is an excellent source of protein and calcium. Since most supermarkets have been carrying yogurt since the early 1960s, only the very unusual forms are sold in health food stores. Their prices usually double the cost of most grocery store varieties. Yogurt was once thought to assist intestinal function by providing certain beneficial bacteria. Control of the intestinal bacteria, however, has been shown not to be very critical or dependent on the intake of yogurt. Yogurt has the same nutritional value as buttermilk, which is considerably less expensive.

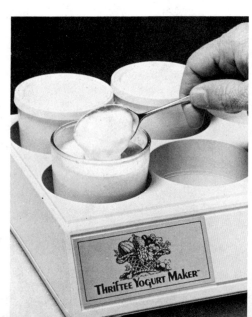

Yogurt is made by adding a mixed culture of two bacteria, Streptococcus thermophilus and Lactobacillus bulgaricus, to pasteurized milk. It can be prepared at home inexpensively in about eight hours. Yogurt is nutritionally similar to milk.

BEE POLLEN

Q. *Will consuming bee pollen tablets help an athlete run faster and farther?*

A. The athletic world can thank the Finns for publicizing bee pollen. It all started in 1972 when Finland's Lasse Viren won the 5,000- and 10,000-meter runs in the Munich Olympics and began buzzing the news about pollen tablets.

When Viren repeated his successes in Montreal in 1976, health food companies decided to make it available at a cost of as much as $45 per pound. The cost is a result of not only its "magical" properties but the way it is gathered. The pollen is gathered by placing wire brushes around the entrances to the bee hives. As the bees obtain nectar from flowers, pollen collects on their bodies. When the bees return to their hives, the wire brushes act as a foot scraper.

This very fine powder is then collected and manufactured into tablets or pellets. Bee pollen in tablet form contains, according to one distributor, all the essential amino acids, vitamins A and most of the B complex, and many trace minerals. There are no magic nutrients in bee pollen that cannot be obtained in conventional, less expensive foods.

Recent research at Louisiana State University conducted by Dr. John C. Wells' group showed that bee pollen has no effect on the performance of runners and swimmers. When confronted with this evidence, a health food distributor noted that the LSU study used bee pollen from France, and not the full-potency pollen from England, which, naturally, he sold! The distributor also said that if an athlete consumed a well-balanced diet, bee pollen would not be beneficial. The supposed value of bee pollen is just another of the many myths that surround the athletic world.

HONEY

Q. *Does the honey sold in the health food stores have any magical properties?*

A. Honey is being sold to health food faddists on the basis of claims ranging from "priceless ingredients," "wonderfully rich in vitamins and minerals," to "it's better for you than sugar." There are dozens of varieties: tupelo, alfalfa, eucalyptus, clover, buckwheat, and orange blossom. And their prices can reach more than $3 per pound.

Chemical analyses of honey show that it does not contain any magical ingredients. It is primarily composed of glucose and fructose with trace amounts of vitamins and minerals. For example, a tablespoon of honey offers .1 milligram of iron and 1 milligram of calcium. So an average young woman could get her iron from 180 tablespoons of honey a day, and her calcium from 1,000 tablespoons. Naturally, honey is not a practical source of these minerals or of any other minerals or vitamins.

VITAMIN B$_{15}$

Q. *Would it be beneficial for health-minded people to consume vitamin B$_{15}$?*

A. Vitamin B$_{15}$, or pangamic acid, is the latest rage in health food stores in the United States. Numerous articles praising this product have appeared in the media. Yet, according to the Food and Drug Administration, "B$_{15}$ is not a vitamin, and no medical or nutritional usefulness for this substance has been established."

In 1943 a patent for a material named pangamic acid was applied for. The material was then trade-named vitamin B$_{15}$. The B$_{15}$ patent application claimed pangamic acid is "a preparation for the immunization of toxic products present in the human or animal system" that has "the property of detoxifying toxic products formed in the human system." The patent application claimed pangamic acid had the property of providing relief for everything from eczema to cancer. Yet the data in the patent application did not support these claims.

The poorly designed studies with conclusions not derived from the data and the studies lacking adequate controls could not produce meaningful positive information.

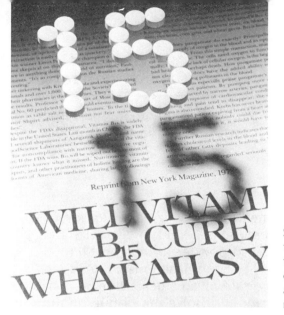

Reprint from New York Magazine, 19__

WILL VITAMIN B₁₅ CURE WHAT AILS Y

Scientific studies show that there is no medical or nutritional usefulness for the so-called "vitamin B₁₅". B₁₅ pills are of no value to fitness-minded people.

The publicized claims of long-term medicinal value for pangamic acid in cancer, alcoholism, emphysema, hepatitis, heart disease, allergies, and diabetes are really testimonial stories rather than the scientifically accepted results of correctly controlled studies.

DESSICATED LIVER

Q. *Would a dessicated liver supplement be helpful to the athlete trying to improve endurance?*

A. Dessicated liver, in pill or powder form, is a good source of vitamin B_{12}. Vitamin B_{12} is vital for protection against pernicious anemia, which results in weakness and loss of energy and endurance. Faddists reasoned that if dessicated liver would prevent a person from getting weak and run-down from anemia, it also would aid in developing endurance. As a result, some athletes have been known to take desiccated liver tablets by the handfuls.

Actually, pernicious anemia is a very rare condition occurring in some people who eat a total vegetarian diet, those who have had their stomach totally removed, and those who cannot absorb the vitamin B_{12} in their diet. Dessicated liver would not help the latter group because they could not absorb the vitamin B_{12} in it. Intramuscular injections of the vitamin would be necessary.

LECITHIN

Q. *Will lecithin prevent men from having heart attacks?*

A. Lecithin, the natural emulsifier found in egg yolks and soybeans, is sold in capsule and powder form at health food stores. It has long been publicized in health magazines as an antidote to high blood cholesterol and heart disease. Evidence shows that lecithin cannot dissolve the plaques in the blood vessels that contribute to heart attacks. Unfortunately, solving the problems associated with high blood cholesterol concentrations and heart attacks is much more complex than a simple feeding of lecithin to the patient.

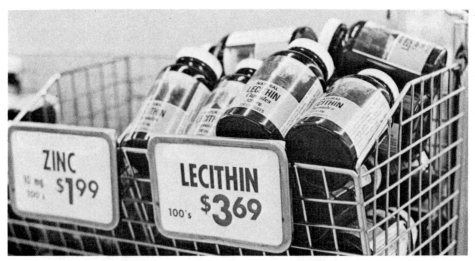

Lecithin, a fat-soluble substance found in many foods and sold in capsule form in health food stores, is not a vitamin or necessary dietary ingredient in any sense.

RAW VEGETABLE JUICES

Q. *Is it healthy to drink several glasses of raw vegetable juice each day?*

A. Carrot juice and other vegetable juices have been promoted using the rationale that the vitamins and minerals contained in these vegetables are essential nutrients, and if a little is good, more is better. In moderate amounts, these juices are not likely to hurt anyone and most of them are quite appealing to the taste buds. Raw vegetable juices, however, are costly and large amounts may provide excessive amounts of liquids and sodium in the diet. Furthermore, the whole fruit or vegetable contributes desirable residue or fiber, which is necessary for normal gastrointestinal function and regularity.

BROWN RICE

Q. *What is brown rice?*

A. Brown rice is just ordinary rice that has not had its outer layers of husk and embryo removed by polishing. It does contain more protein and vitamins. than unenriched white rice, but the difference is small enough to be unimportant unless rice forms a major portion of a person's diet. Some extremists advocate eating practically nothing but brown rice and other grains—a diet that is grossly deficient in many nutrients and even dangerous. Several people have in fact starved to death following such a diet.

GARLIC

Q. *Does the garlic sold in health food stores have any magical powers?*

A. Garlic is a plant whose strong-smelling bulbs are used for seasoning meats, salads, and other foods. Raw garlic and garlic oil capsules, however, are often claimed to purify the blood, reduce high blood pressure, and prevent cancer, diph-

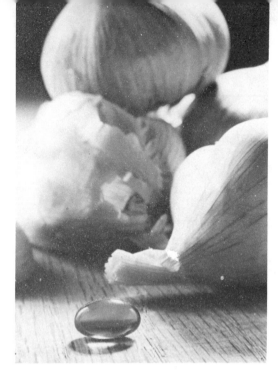

There is no magical nutrient in garlic or a garlic oil capsule that is not found in a balanced diet.

theria, pneumonia, and symptoms of aging. Eleanor Roosevelt even believed that she kept her memory sharp by eating three chocolate-covered garlic balls every morning at breakfast. None of these claims has been proved by scientific studies. While garlic does contain some vitamins and minerals, it would have to be consumed in very large quantities to contribute significantly to a person's daily requirements.

EXOTIC FOODS

Q. What about the large number of exotic foods that are displayed in health food stores? Should a health-minded person consider consuming them?

A. Many people are becoming interested in exotic foods. Should sesame seeds be on the dining room table, or cod liver oil in the pantry? Will avocado oil clear the complexion? Which tea is best for health—buckthorn, mullein leaf, slippery elm, wormwood, or sassafras? These exotic products go on and on. And each product is supposed to provide a specific benefit for health, according to the faddist.

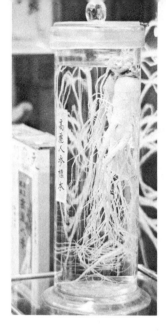

Ginseng root is currently promoted as an aphrodisiac. Anyone considering trying it should take heed. Ginseng contains a variety of potentially toxic chemicals. Among its toxic effects are diarrhea, skin eruptions, insomnia, nervousness, and severe mental confusion.

Medical authorities and nutrition scientists who are not earning a living from the sale of health foods seem to agree about answers to these questions. The individual should stay away from exotic and obscure food products unless he knows exactly what they are and what they will do. Furthermore, an individual should not be afraid to seek professional advice when questions or problems arise.

HEALTH FOOD WRITERS

Q. *Popular health food author, the late Adelle Davis, has written that "almost every American suffers from nutritional deficiencies." She has pointed to highly processed, devitalized foods as a prime cause of modern health problems. Is this true?*

A. Such indictments are ancient. Medicine, however, cannot trace plagues of serious illness in modern America to processed foods. Physicians continue to wonder where all these food-sickened people are. And where is the proof that specific illnesses are caused by the food we eat? Can health food faddists really believe that through ignorance, indifference, or conspiracy, hundreds of thousands of physicians and scientists are suppressing the real causes, cures, and preventions of disease? The plain fact is that national health surveys find the vast majority of nutrients to be plentiful in American food.

"The real need is for Americans to understand their nutritional needs," says Dr. Roslyn Alfin-Slater of the University of California at Los Angeles, "and to know the role each food plays in filling these needs. Ultimately, such knowledge is the surest defense against poor nutrition as a health problem. Good food for a good diet is all around us. We need only learn to choose."

HEALTH FOODS NO PANACEA

Q. *What type of people buy health foods?*

A. According to James Trager, three basic groups are interested in health foods: (1) people motivated by a simple desire for good food, (2) people concerned about environmental decay from persistent chemical pesticides and herbicides, and (3) people who have anxieties about their appearance and physical well-being, which they link to what they eat. The third group, which includes many athletes, is by far the largest of the three.

Members of these groups frequently testify that they feel just "wonderful" as a result of eating this food or taking that pill. The alleged benefit of health foods may be in the *faith* that the buyer puts in these foods. This psychological benefit or placebo effect should not be sold short.

No doubt much of the faith in health foods is developed from the positive encouragement of the so-called "nutrition counselor" behind the cash register. Such counselors thrive because customers need them. Ignorant consumers cry for positive advice and remedies to their problems. The danger of this advice lies in the fact that most of the nutrition counselors are self-trained and have no formal background in nutrition or medicine. Yet they dispense information that the customer takes as the gospel truth! Most of this advice is simply ridiculous and unjustified. "How to succeed without trying" seems to be the cry of most people in trouble and they are eager to believe any promise of cure, no matter how ridiculous it may sound, as long as it does not demand self-discipline or a change in habits upon which they have become dependent.

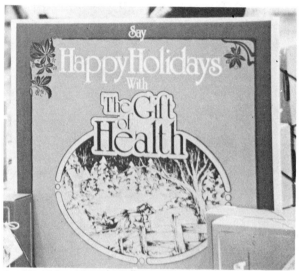

A gift of health makes good advertising sense during the holiday season. Unfortunately, health is much more complex than giving and receiving a gift from a health food store.

Often people with nutrient deficiencies or unusual nutrient requirements cannot be safely self-diagnosed or self-treated. Pills should not be substituted for meals. Furthermore, it is difficult for the layman who is searching for an answer to tell the difference between useful recommendations and the sales pitch of a product. A person may waste money taking unprescribed vitamins and mineral supplements and do himself no harm, since the excess is usually excreted. Overdoses of vitamins A and D, however, can be harmful and the prolonged intake of excessive amounts of energy sources, protein, and various minerals can produce serious damage to health and well-being.

The products sold in health food stores are not more nutritious than products sold at local supermarkets. In fact, they are much more expensive and it is often difficult to be certain a person is getting the product that the label claims. Fitness-minded individuals should not be misled about the power of health food products.

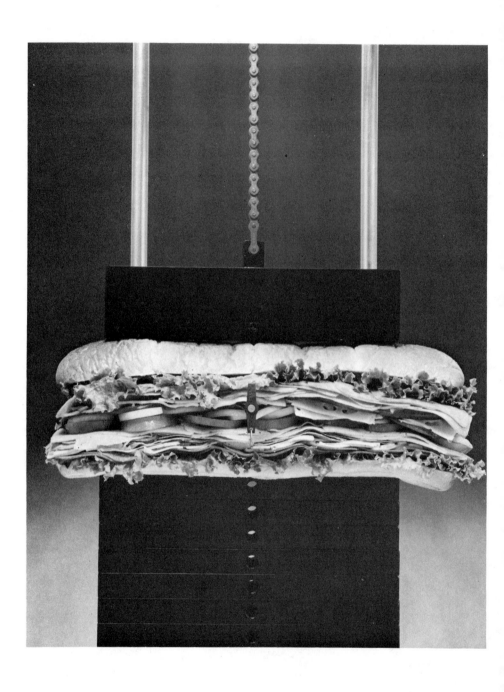

IV.

DYNAMICS OF NUTRITION WITH EXERCISE

15

losing body fat

BODY FAT DEFINED

Q. *What is body fat?*

A. Chemically speaking, fat is composed of 6% proteins, 72% lipids, and 22% water. Because of the high concentration of lipids, a pound of fat contains 3,500 calories, or about six times the calories as an equal amount of muscle tissue.

Seen under the microscope, fat tissue looks like a bubble bath. The globules are grouped together with stringy intercellular glue and streaked with narrow filaments of connective tissue, blood vessels, and nerves. This network of fat cells is designed to provide a versatile, living inner tube, inflatable or deflatable as required, with minimum stress and strain to both the skin on the outside that encloses it and the viscera on the inside that it encloses.

TYPES OF BODY FAT

Q. *Are there different types of body fat?*

246

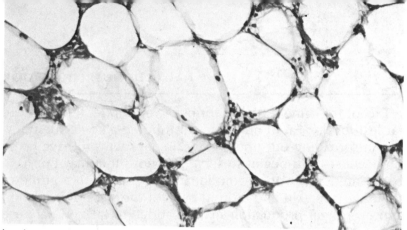

A microscopic view of human fat tissue resembles a bubble bath. (Photo by Nellie Wiggins)

A. Yes, there are three classifications of body fat:

1. Subcutaneous fat is fat that lies in layers directly under the skin.

2. Depot fat is inherited fat deposited in certain areas of the body.

3. Essential fat is fat that cushions and protects many vital organs of the body.

About 50% of fat stored by the average human body is subcutaneous, 40% is depot, and 10% is essential. A person can reduce subcutaneous and depot fat but not essential fat.

FUNCTION OF FAT

Q. *What is the function of fat in the human body?*

A. The primary function of body fat is the long-term storage of fuel. The use of fat for fuel did not begin with humans. Almost from the beginning of life on earth, fat has had a biological role to play as fuel storage for moving organisms. Larval forms of certain insects may carry 90% of their weight in lipid form. Locusts and monarch butterflies prepare for long-distance migrations through preflight feeding and fat depositing that can last for several days. Before migrating, birds may fatten themselves by 25% in a week. Several species of fish, notably salmon and sharks, are recognized for their lipid reserves, which provide energy for their long-distance swims.

Except for camels, higher forms of vertebrates tend to store fat less locally. Fat in humans is distributed all over the body. But in spreading out under the skin, fat seems to have taken on new uses and begins to serve functions that may not have been intended in the evolutionary process. With a girdle of fat under the skin and around parts of the viscera, insulation and even heat production may be added to fat's primary use as an energy storage depot.

UNATTRACTIVE FAT

Q. *If fat is a necessary part of the human body, why has it received such bad publicity in recent times?*

A. In the last 40 years it has become popular among physicians, insurance underwriters, psychotherapists, and fashion designers to attack obesity as a common enemy. Over the years campaigns mustered in this cause have raised legions of specialists and specialties. A recent poll showed that 90% of the public does not like the way it looks. Americans, in fact, spend billions of dollars annually on diet and weight-reducing drugs, fad diet books, reducing machines, and health courses.

The bountiful supply of food in this country makes the ability to store fat no longer a lifesaving necessity. If anything, actuarial tables suggest that it may be just the opposite.

Insurance studies that ushered in a new world in body images for Americans were first published in 1912. As an indirect result, we are now taught that being overfat increases our chances of dying of heart disease, diabetes, and nephritis. There has also been the extra burden of psychological guilt produced by the fashion, sports, and fitness industries. Few people want to date a fat person, do business with a butterball executive, or play tennis with an obese partner.

EVALUATION OF BODY FAT

Q. *How serious is the obesity problem in the United States?*

A. The most recent figures published by the insurance

companies suggested that almost 50% of the adult women in the United States are seriously overweight. Figures for adult males run a close second. If an obesity rate of 50% seems high, Americans can take some comfort from the recent data released by the Baden-Wurttemburg State Medical Association, which estimates the German obesity rate for both sexes at close to 70%.

Experience has shown, however, that even if an average person is at a correct body weight for his height, he is still likely to be too fat for playing sports in the most efficient manner. And he is probably too fat for his optimum level of physical fitness. Exercise physiology clinics that routinely measure and evaluate body fat note that only once in a great while do they actually find an adult who is too lean. More than 99% of the people they measure are too fat.

"PINCH" TEST

Q. *How does a person know if he is overfat?*
A. Obesity has been defined as starting anywhere from

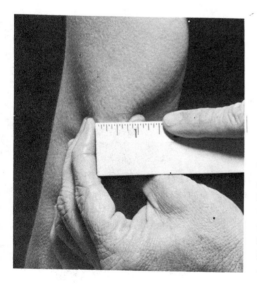

The pinch test can be used to estimate percentage of body fat. Grasp the skin on the back of the upper arm and measure its thickness with a ruler. This photograph shows a skinfold thickness of 3/4 inch, an indication of between 18 and 23% body fat for this woman.

10–25% above actuarially "normal" weights for a given height. At best, however, the use of such tables and percentages have proven only reasonably correct. At worst, they provide merely interesting guesswork.

An individual can obtain a fair estimate of his body fat by using the "pinch test." The following procedure applies both to men and women:

Directions

1. Have a friend do the pinching and measuring. A person cannot measure his own skinfold.

2. Let the right arm hang down to the side.

3. Locate the skinfold site on the back of the upper arm midway between the shoulder and the elbow.

4. Grasp a vertical fold of skin between the thumb and first finger. Pull the skin and fat away from the arm. Make sure the fold does not include any muscle, just skin and fat. Practice pinching and pulling the skin until there is no muscle included.

5. Measure with a ruler the thickness of the skinfold to the nearest one-quarter inch. Be sure to measure the distance between the thumb and the finger. Sometimes the top of the skinfold is thicker than the distance between the thumb and finger. To avoid this, make sure the top of the skinfold is level with the top of the thumb. Do not press the ruler against the skinfold. This will flatten it out and make it appear thicker than it really is.

6. Take the two separate measures of skinfold thickness, releasing the skin between each measure, to determine the average thickness.
Skinfold #1 _____ Skinfold #2 _____ Average skinfold _____

7. Estimate percentage of body fat from the following chart.

Percentage of Fat—Men			Percentage of Fat—Women		
Skinfold (inches) Thickness		Percentage	Skinfold (inches) Thickness		Percentage
¼	=	5–9	¼	=	8–13
½	=	9–13	½	=	13–18
¾	=	13–18	¾	=	18–23
1	=	18–22	1	=	23–28
1¼	=	22–27	1¼	=	28–33

Most Americans have more than 25% of their body weight in fat. Athletes have a smaller percentage of fat than nonathletes. An ideal amount of body fat for most men is below 12%. The average female interested in a slender figure should strive for less than 18% body fat.

CLIMATE AND BODY FAT

Q. *It seems that people up North are fatter than people down South. Is this correct? Why?*

A. Generally speaking, this is a correct observation. Over centuries and centuries, populations have adapted to their geographical locations. Studies have shown that the predominant physical type within any given region will be one that is best adapted to the climate. The odds of blond hair being found in a sunny tropical climate are low. Fair-skinned people do not adjust well to hot, open environments unless they spend most of their time indoors. The gene pool in such a climate will contain few genes for blondness but many for dark skin and hair.

Conversely, in colder countries, children with light skin and hair are able to extract more vitamin D from sunlight than can their dark-haired brothers and sisters. Thus, it is the blonds who thrive. Over the centuries, colder areas of the world will tend to accumulate genes for blondness and genes for dark hair will gradually tend to become scarce.

Both heat and cold are stressful to the human body. In fact, there seems to be a strong relationship between body weight and annual mean temperature. The colder the mean temperature, the heavier the body weight. The warmer the mean temperature, the lighter the body weight.

The relative leanness of warm-dwelling people, and the relative fatness of cold-dwelling people, can be traced back to a period roughly 18,000 to 25,000 years ago. In the cold regions of that time period, the ability to store surplus fat under the skin on the least possible total food intake may have made the difference between life and death.

Central heating, air conditioning, and mass production of warm clothing serve to minimize the individual's exposure to environmental extremes. Even so, scientists can document the extraordinary degree that the modern American still seems programmed by blueprints laid down by our Ice Age ancestors.

Among white Americans, obesity is lowest in people of British, Irish, or "Old American" origins, and slightly higher in people of Scandinavian and Germanic ancestry. The fattest Americans of all tend to be people of Balto-Ugraic, Central Slav, and Soviet-Russian ancestry.

There is a striking correlation between body build and an individual's city or state of origin within the United States. The leanest Americans come from the southeastern United States. The fattest ones come from the Mid-Atlantic states and the Midwest.

GENETICS AND FAT CELLS

Q. *Are some people naturally inclined to be fat?*

A. Genetic factors certainly play a role in a person's potential fatness and leanness. While almost all people can get fatter or leaner with proper diet and exercise, there are definite limits.

There are two limiting factors on the amount of fat a person can store. First is the number of fat cells the individual is born with or acquires within the first few months of life. Second is the size of each fat cell. Overfeeding results in a ballooning of each cell to several times its original size. The actual number of fat cells in a person's reserve depot remains the same throughout his life and seems to be determined at or slightly after birth.

Dr. Jean Mayer, President of Tufts University, studied the inherited tendencies of fatness while he was professor of nutrition at Harvard University. Dr. Mayer estimates that if both parents are obese, 80% of the children will follow suit. If one parent is fat, the risk of obesity in children is 40%. If both parents are lean, the chance of fatness, he feels, is only 7%. What seems to be important is the *tendency* to fatness.

Thus our tendency toward fatness or our number of fat cells is determined early in life. But our fatness or leanness within this limitation can still be a matter of choice—a choice primarily related to diet and exercise.

The tendency toward fatness and leanness is a genetic characteristic. Children with obese parents have a much greater probability of being overfat than do children with lean parents. (Photo by Ellington Darden)

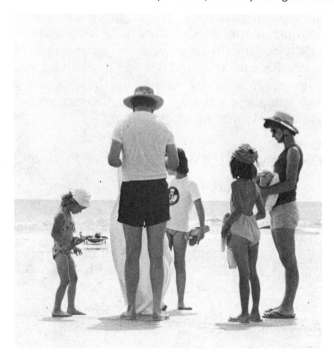

PREGNANCY AND FAT DEPOSITION

Q. *Is pregnancy fattening?*

A. Women all over the world seem to be designed to gain extra fat during pregnancy, no matter how fat or lean they may have been to begin with. Research has shown that the average weight gain from the beginning of the first trimester until the end of pregnancy is 27.5 pounds, of which about 20% is fat.

The reason for this weight gain is probably to make allowances for a certain caloric reserve against the stress of childbirth. A margin of safety has been built into the system in the form of the mother's own fat reserves. Nature has arranged matters so that, even without another person to provision her, the mother and child can survive, at least for a while, on the mother's fat stores.

Recent research suggests that there may have to be a minimum of fat tissue before adolescent girls can start to menstruate and to conceive and bear children. All over the world, girls of every culture show a sudden weight spurt at puberty.

Before puberty girls have 10–15% more fat than do boys. But at the end of adolescence they have twice as much fat as boys. Girls tend to gain an average of 35.2 pounds of stored fat between the ages of 9 and 15. Some scientists even think this additional fat is programmed into the mother's body to ensure the species' continuity even in the face of short-term famine, social isolation, or abandonment.

HORMONES AND FATNESS

Q. *How important are hormones in fatness and leanness?*

A. Hormones are very important. Male sex hormones contribute to leanness and female sex hormones contribute to fatness. This is one reason why obese women have a more difficult time losing fat and keeping it off than do obese men.

Estrogen, a female hormone, seems to have an affinity for

fat cells in certain parts of the body. Fat breasts represent sites of high estrogen receptivity. So do the buttocks and hips.

Estrogen is also related to pregnancy. As pregnancy progresses, so does estrogen production.

Another female hormone, progesterone, is secreted generously throughout pregnancy but especially so toward term. It is progesterone that is credited with the monthly weight gain that troubles some women toward the end of their menstrual cycles.

INHERITED PATTERNS OF FAT DISTRIBUTION

Q. *What are some inherited patterns of fat distribution?*

A. Just as different families and different races have charac-

Many men store much of their fat around the navel area. Bob Smart of Seattle, Washington is an example of an individual who decided to do something about his overfat condition. On March 26, 1981, Bob weighed 208 pounds. He was put on a 1,500-calorie-a-day, well-balanced diet and began training three times per week on Nautilus equipment. Eight weeks later, on May 21, 1981, he weighed 180 pounds. Bob Smart, at 57 years of age, had the discipline, motivation, and patience to lose 28 pounds in 56 days. (Photos by Ellington Darden)

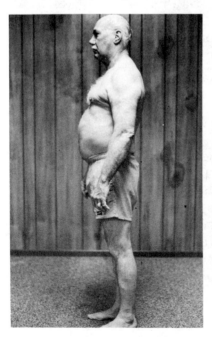 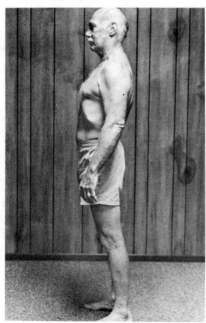

teristic heights, coloring, and nose shapes, they may have characteristic patterns of fat distribution. Perhaps the best known racial variant is that of the African Hottentot and Bushman. If the women become obese, the bulk of fat is deposited as a great mound around the buttocks. The mound may actually grow to the size of a large watermelon while the woman remains relatively lean over the rest of her body.

Hormones also influence the distribution of body fat. Androgens and estrogens are largely responsible for the differences in the way men and women deposit fat. The breasts, for example, are mostly fat, not glandular tissue as many people imagine, and estrogens are particularly responsible for this fat distribution.

Men, as they get older, tend to deposit their fat more frontally than do women. Women tend to deposit their fat more on the back of the body. This is true not only for that percentage of fat that accumulates in their buttocks, but also for the lower part of their backs as well. Another genetic difference is that men tend to deposit more of their fat on the trunk rather than on the arms and legs, as women do. Male fat is usually truncal fat as well as frontal.

Much of the adipose tissue that a man accumulates on his front will be concentrated in the area above the navel in the low-slung "beer belly." Fat women usually concentrate their truncal fat below the navel and over the hips.

LOSING FAT SLOWLY

Q. *Is there a quick and easy way to lose excessive body fat?*

A. It is virtually impossible to lose body fat quickly and easily. Almost anyone can lose five or ten pounds of body weight on a short-term basis. The sad part is that unless it is done slowly, most of the weight loss will be water that comes from the muscles and organs rather than fat stores. What counts is losing weight permanently and making sure that the weight loss is fat. This requires discipline, motivation, and patience.

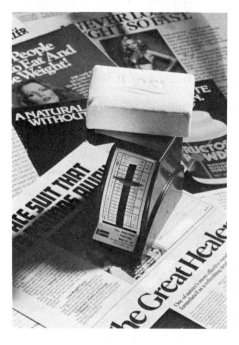

A person adhering to a reducing diet should expect to lose about $3\frac{1}{2}$ ounces of fat a day, or an amount equal to the size of an average bar of soap. Contrary to what weight-loss advertisements promote, it is impossible for the average dieter to lose fat quickly.

ADVERTISING OFFERING FAST WEIGHT LOSS

Q. *What about all the ads in popular magazines that promise fast results?*

A. A large percentage of advertising in popular magazines offering fast weight loss is myth, half truths, or outright lies. Many of them involve dangerous practices. Some of the more popular ones peddling miraculous ways to lose fat have been:

Tone-O-Matic: A company that claims that by simply wearing their Tone-O-Matic weighted belt an individual can "whittle inches off his waist." A useless gadget, according to the Federal Trade Commission, which also says that by wearing the weighted belt some individuals "could physically injure themselves."

Relaxacizor: An electrical device that transmits current to the muscles through contact pads strapped on the body. Actually, the muscle movements are too small to consume enough energy to cause a noticeable reduction in fat. Doctors believe these machines can be dangerous to the heart and other organs that can respond to electrical stimuli.

Vibrating belts: A mechanical vibrating belt may relax a

person and make him feel better, but it certainly will not remove fat. Fat cannot be shaken, tickled, beaten, or stroked from the body.

Rubber clothes: These clothes, which range from belts, shorts, and shirts to full outfits, are supposed to make a person sweat off the fat and inches. Any weight lost is merely a result of dehydration, which is quickly replaced when the individual quenches his thirst. Since fat contains only a small percentage of water, little of the water comes from the person's body fat.

Sauna wraps: Sauna wrap is a tape that has been soaked in a "secret" solution. The body, or the specific part a person wants reduced, is wrapped with this tape. The person then sits in a sauna bath for thirty minutes and the secret solution supposedly draws the excess fat from the body. Again, fat cannot be sweated out of the body.

Cellulite remedies: Cellulite is a trade word supposedly connoting a unique type of fat that can be removed only by a costly and elaborate program. The American Medical Association has issued a statement calling cellulite a hoax and denouncing its remedies as economic exploitation.

Over-the-counter drugs: Despite the efforts of the pharmaceutical industry, no satisfactory fat-reduction drug has been developed. Nobody will lose fat simply by consuming a certain capsule, tablet, or pill. In the opinion of many physicians, claims for most over-the-counter weight loss and appetite control products are nonsense or lies. At best, some offer temporary suppression of appetite. They should be withdrawn from the market.

CONSUMER PROTECTION

Q. *Can't the government do more to stop misleading advertisements?*

A. The Food and Drug Administration, the Federal Trade Commission, and the Post Office Department deal to some extent in diet and exercise gimmicks. Several years ago the Post Office Department set out to prove that the Sauna Belt* did not do what it claimed to do. They particularly did not agree with the idea that the belt could reduce dimensions without reducing body weight.

Testifying in court, the scientist from the government noted: "There is no really successful way of reducing the waistline without reducing body weight as a whole. The inert fatty substance cannot be in any way increased or decreased in volume by massage, compression, or exercise."

The Sauna Belt people, however, came up with their own expert, a professor of physiology at a small university in California. This professor insisted that spot reduction had taken place, explaining "it was a redistribution of the fat layer." He went on to say that there are *mysterious* things happening under the belt.

To make the story short, the postal authorities lost the case. As a result, hundreds of thousands of Sauna Belts, or variations, have been sold to the public since then.

In the long run, it looks like a losing battle for the protectors of consumer rights. Although the criminal statute provides for heavy penalties, courts and juries will not convict unless the essential element of *intent to defraud* is abundantly present. It is not enough to prove that claims for a product are true or false. It must be proved that the promoter knew them to be false. This is the crucial issue. The defendant need explain nothing. He is innocent and remains so until the court overcomes this presumption.

The clever promoter, therefore, can often advertise almost anything he wants to and get away with it for a surprisingly long period of time.

The individual must realize that no one is going to protect him from untrue advertisements and their products. He must rely on his own judgment to guard against fitness frauds. Scientific evidence clearly shows that there is no quick and easy way to lose body fat.

---

*An inflatible, rubberized belt that is placed around the waist before exercising and left on for a time after the exercise to let the midsection "steam away excess pounds and inches."

CELLULITE

Q. *The earlier comment about cellulite is confusing. Why isn't it a special type of fat that is very difficult to remove?*

A. There is nothing special about cellulite. But perhaps a bit more explanation will help.

The relationship among the skin, the fat, and the underlying muscles and fascia are rather distinctive in human beings. Other species have fur, feathers, and certain blood-shunting devices in their bag of cold-weather tricks. But we humans have virtually nothing between us and the elements except fat and skin. This may be one of the reasons that fat adheres so stubbornly to our underlying fascia.

It is this adhesiveness that accounts for the kind of dimpling effect that has been dubbed *cellulite*. The term has been applied to the puckering or dimpling of fat that occurs in the buttocks and thighs of overfat and usually middle-aged women. Cellulite has become such a common word that it would be pointless to try to remove it from the dieter's vocabulary. Although there is no such word medically, the condition it refers to is one that can and does exist.

What apparently happens in cellulite is that the ribbons of connective tissue, which serve as pouches for large groups of fat cells in sort of a honeycomb arrangement under the skin, have lost their elasticity and shrink with age. The overlying skin attached to these fibers then contracts. If the size of the fat cells encased in them does not shrink to match, a kind of overall dimpling occurs on the surface of the skin.

The cure for this is simply to reduce the size of the empouched fat by dieting. The individual's goal should be to shrink the fat cells inside the pockets of connective tissue down to the limits of the shrunken connective fibers.

SEARCHING FOR A FOOLPROOF WAY

Q. *Is there a foolproof way to lose fat and keep it off permanently?*

A. There is no foolproof way to lose and keep fat off. In one scientifically conducted clinical fat-reduction program,

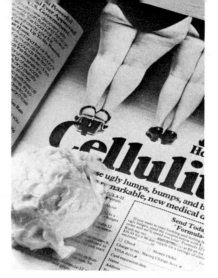

Whether it is lumpy or bumpy, dimpled or pocked, thick or thin, fat is still fat. And all fat is removed from the body in the same way: by causing the fat cells to shrink gradually as a result of the caloric intake being lower than the caloric output.

only 10% of the patients managed to maintain their original weight losses after one year. At two years this figure had dropped to 6%. After a five-year period this ratio had dwindled to less than 1%.

The highest success rates for any groups were for male volunteers who were members of an Anti-Coronary Club program in New York City. The men enrolled in the program were a high-risk group in terms of age, lifestyle, and eating habits. The results of this study program reflect the life-and-death rationale attending the program itself.

In the light of this information, however, one thing remains clear: There is no way to become fat without eating too much food for the body to handle. And there is no way to become lean without eating less food than the body needs to store.

DIETING

Q. *What type of diet is recommended to lose fat?*

A. A well-balanced, lower-calorie diet is the choice of the nutritional and medical professions. It should produce a small, weekly amount of fat loss—without producing long-lasting hunger.

Hunger, in all shapes, sizes, and degrees, is the dieter's ghost. The object in long-haul fat reduction is to learn to cheat that hunger as gracefully and as intelligently as possible. The table on the next page is a simple guideline for losing fat.

Dietary Guidelines for Losing Fat
(Sample Diets)

Food	For 1,200 Calories Daily	For 1,500 Calories Daily	Notes
Meat Group	3 small servings (or a total of 7 ounces cooked weight)	3 small servings (or a total of 7 ounces cooked weight)	Choose lean, well-trimmed meats: beef, veal, lamb, pork. Poultry and fish should have skin removed. One egg can be substituted for 1 serving of meat.
Milk Group	2 cups fortified	2 cups whole milk	Two cups milk means two 8-ounce measuring cups.
Fruits and Vegetables Group	4 servings	4 servings	One fruit serving = 1 medium fruit, 2 small fruits, 1/2 banana, 1/4 cantaloupe, 10–12 grapes or cherries, 1 cup fresh berries or 1/2 cup fresh, canned or frozen unsweetened fruit or fruit juice. Include one citrus fruit or other good source of vitamin C daily. One vegetable serving = 1/2 cup cooked or 1 cup raw leafy vegetable. Include one dark green or deep yellow vegetable or other good source of vitamin A at least every other day.
Bread and Cereal Group	4 servings	5 servings	One serving = 1 slice bread; 1 small dinner roll; 1/2 cup cooked cereal, noodles, macaroni, spaghetti, rice, cornmeal; 1 ounce (about 1 cup) ready-to-eat unsweetened iron-fortified cereal.
Other foods	1 serving	3 servings	One serving = 1 teaspoon butter, margarine, or oil; 6 nuts; 2 teaspoons salad dressing; or 35 calories or less of another food.

An important principle in losing body fat is strict adherence to a diet that is restricted in calories but balanced in nutrient content. The preceding chart is nutritionally balanced and based on the Four Basic Food Groups: meat, milk, fruits and vegetables, and breads and cereals.

Most people should begin by following the guidelines for 1,500 calories a day. Gradually, within four to six weeks, they should progress to 1,200 calories a day. On this plan, they should notice a slow and steady loss of body weight.

For those individuals who want more stringent dietary guidelines, a fourteen-day, 1,000 calorie-a-day diet is listed in Appendix C.

SCARSDALE DIET

Q. *What could be wrong with using the popular Scarsdale Diet for reducing body fat?*

A. The Scarsdale Diet is a high-protein, low-carbohydrate, low-calorie pattern that has appeared many times in the past. The late Dr. Herman Tarnover, the creator of the diet, prescribed a rigid, two-week meal schedule. Breakfast is always the same: one-half grapefruit, one slice of bread, and black coffee or tea. Lunches include foods such as coldcuts, low-fat cottage cheese, eggs, vegetables, and sometimes dry toast. Dinners include foods such as chicken, fish, and vegetables. Strict adherence to the program promises a pound a day in weight loss.

It should be pointed out, however, that there is a big difference between weight loss and fat loss. Only three to four ounces of fat can be lost daily. The weight that is lost from the Scarsdale Diet comes primarily from water loss and depletion of vital organs.

Low-carbohydrate diets have obvious repercussions for the fitness-minded person. The body has a specific need for carbohydrates as a source of energy for the brain and other specialized functions. The normal adult requires at least 400 carbohydrate calories daily. If these are not provided in the diet, they must be derived from the breakdown of protein and fat. When the body has to resort to the breakdown of protein for energy, the primary source is muscle tissue.

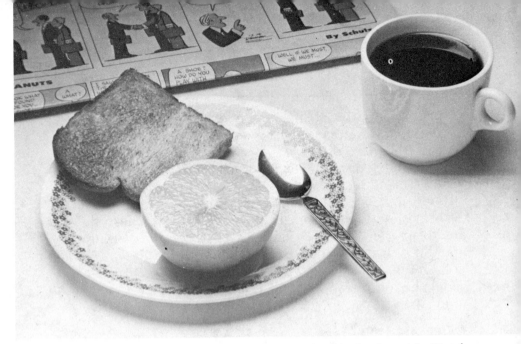

It is almost impossible for a person to stick with the Scarsdale Diet for more than several weeks. The Scarsdale Diet and other high-protein, low-carbohydrate diets are not recommended for fitness-minded people.

As the rate of fat metabolism accelerates, ketosis occurs. Ketosis occurs when water is extracted from the tissues in order to eliminate the toxic substances created as fat is metabolized. This stresses the kidneys and leads to the loss of valuable minerals.

Loss of muscle mass is clearly an undesirable effect for an active person, but the depletion of water, minerals, and the accompanying fatigue also have serious consequences. Water is needed for the control of body temperature, for proper functioning of enzymes, for digestion and metabolism, for elimination of nitrogen wastes, and for transportation and utilization of nutrients. When more than 2–3% of the body's water is lost, physical performance suffers. Calcium loss may cause muscle weakness and, in some cases, spasms. And finally, lowered glycogen stores reduce endurance and cause early exhaustion during activity.

People who wish to go on this diet should understand these facts.

MAYO DIET

Q. *What about the Mayo Diet, which concentrates on eggs and grapefruit?*

A. The Mayo Clinic indignantly disclaims any connection with this diet. The enzymes found in grapefruit are claimed somehow to dissolve calories by acting as a catalyst to increase the fat-burning process. This diet, which advises an individual to eat plenty of eggs and meat, is high in saturated fats and cholesterol. Grapefruit is a nutritious low-calorie food that tends to satisfy the appetite rather well, as do most other fresh fruits. But nothing found in grapefruit is capable of dissolving fat.

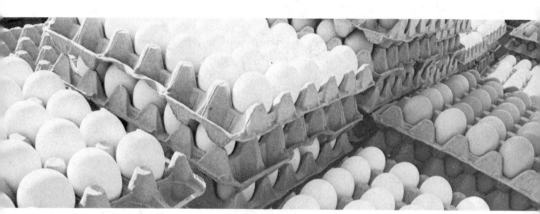

Eggs are included in many fad diets because they are rich in proteins and fats and contain almost no carbohydrates. Most of the weight lost initially on a low-carbohydrate diet comes from the body's water stores, rather than fat stores.

SKIPPING MEALS

Q. *Is it okay to skip a meal occasionally?*

A. Many people who do skip meals have the tendency to nibble later on or overeat at the next meal. They actually may end up consuming more calories for the day. Most serious dieters should adhere to at least three small balanced meals per day.

TRICKING HUNGER

Q. *Are there ways to "trick" hunger when dieting?*

A. Yes, there are certain ideas that can be applied to bring the feeling of hunger under control. Three physiological subsystems are involved in hunger: the brain, the gut, and the endocrine system.

The first line of defense against the false hunger of appetite is the brain, or more specifically, the hypothalamus. Signals that we as dieters can inject into the hypothalamus include cues about body temperature, blood and tissue oxygen levels, tissue water supplies, and glucose supplies.

Perhaps the easiest to manipulate is heat. One way of persuading the brain that the body is being fed is to turn up body heat. Body heat can be increased by eating or drinking something hot or by deliberately setting out to raise skin temperature by putting on extra clothes and moving into a warm environment.

Another way to trick the unfed hypothalamus is to persuade it that there is more oxygen in the tissues than is actually there. If a person feels hungry, he should do some exercise.

The time it takes various food components to pass through the gut can also be used to advantage. The ideal meal plan for someone with an ungovernable appetite is to start the meal with something sweet and follow it with a salad, then eat the rest of the meal.

Dieters who have trouble keeping their appetite in check at parties and gala dinners should prediet rather than postdiet. If a person must overeat, he should do it on an empty stomach.

The second line of defense against hunger is the gut. One way to trick the gut into feeling fed is to eat large amounts of low-calorie foods. This can make the dieter feel so full that he does not want food. Salads and vegetables are good for this purpose. So are soups and cereals. And the hotter the food, the better.

The common advice to drink plenty of water while on a diet is appropriate. Not only does water make a person feel full, but whatever works to preserve fat stores in the body seems closely calibrated to whatever it is that conserves water.

Special attention should also be given to carbohydrate intake. Fat burns best and fastest in the presence of carbohydrates, and the dieter's own lean tissue is at risk when there is no starch or sugar coming into the system to provide fuel for burning fat. At least 50% of a well-balanced, fat-reducing diet should be in the form of carbohydrates.

IMPORTANCE OF EXERCISE IN FAT REDUCTION

Q. *How important is the role of exercise in fat reduction?*

A. A low-calorie diet does result in weight loss. Careful studies show that some of this weight loss comes not from body fat but from the muscles, vital organs, and extracellular fluid. Loss of protein from these vital cells and organs is difficult to avoid with even small reduction of the caloric intake of an inactive person. This problem is readily overcome if a firm diet is combined with increased exercise. Additional calories are used, physical appearance and condition are improved, and activity helps quell hunger pangs.

For a dieter to get the most out of an exercise program, the exercises must be properly selected and properly performed. Just any group of exercises will not do the job.

The exercise should involve all major muscles. It should involve full-range movement, and it should be progressive. Nautilus machines meet these requirements well.

Muscles that are properly strengthened require more calories at *rest*. This is a very important fact.

The real problem in most cases of obesity begins with how many calories a person uses when he is not doing anything. Caloric use at rest decreases as an individual gets older. In other words, if he eats the same number of calories he ate

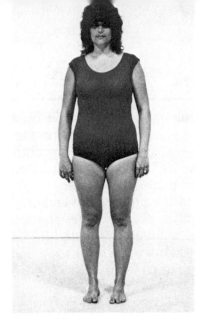 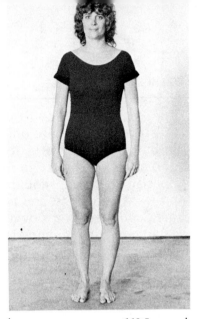

138 pounds ⟶ 3 months later ⟶ 119.5 pounds

Carlene Merry, a 28-year-old mother of two children, began a fat-loss and exercise program on June 11, 1980. Her body weight was 138 pounds and her percentage of body fat according to skinfold calipers was 28.5%. Carlene reduced her calories to 1,200 a day. She trained on Nautilus equipment twice a week. Three months later, Carlene's body weight was 119.5, a reduction of 18.5 pounds. Her percentage of body fat was 16.5, which amounted to an actual loss of 19.61 pounds of fat. Her lean muscle mass increased 1.11 pounds and her strength on 10 Nautilus exercises improved 44.5%. (Photos by Ellington Darden)

when he was younger and did the same amount of physical activity, he would still get fat.

Muscle cells are active cells. They are busy all the time. Fat cells are fairly inactive. They do not have nearly as many blood vessels in them as do active muscle cells.

As we get older, we tend to lose muscle cells. One reason for this is failure to maintain physical activity of the type that strengthens the large muscles.

A proper treatment program for obesity, therefore, should not only decrease calorie intake and increase physical activity, but should also include measures to maintain the resting energy turnover by the body. This simply means that a dieter needs to strengthen his muscles and keep them strong through proper exercise. And this is true for both men and women.

How to Take Before-and-After Photographs. Individuals who are serious about a fat-loss and exercise program can have a visual record of their progress by following these directions:

- Wear a snug bathing suit or leotard and have full-length photographs taken against an uncluttered background. Do not try to pose. Stand perfectly relaxed for three pictures—front, side, and back views.

- Have two prints made of each negative. On the back of each photograph in both sets write the date and body weight. File one set for safekeeping.

- Select the least attractive photograph of the remaining set, the one that shows the most fat, and carry it around in a billfold or pocketbook. Look at it often, especially before meals and before retiring.

- Adhere strictly to the fat-loss and exercise program in this book.

- Repeat the picture-taking session every month. Compare the photographs with the preceding sets.

- Use the before-and-after photographs as a reminder of the previous state of fatness and as motivation for continued fat loss.

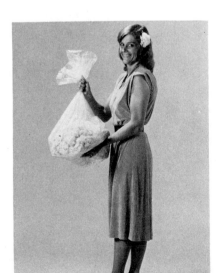

Losing 20 pounds of body fat can make a drastic difference in a person's appearance. To illustrate this concept, Carlene Merry is shown holding a plastic bag that contains 20 pounds of beef fat.

NAUTILUS WORKOUTS

Q. *What is the recommended Nautilus exercise program for a person on a low-calorie diet?*

A. The important thing for a dieter to remember is to exercise all the major muscles at least twice a week. Any of the workouts listed on pages 127 and 128 of *The Nautilus Book* could be selected. Or the following routines may be used:

Routine A	*Routine B*
1. Hip and Back	1. Hip Abduction
2. Leg Extension	2. Hip Abduction
3. Leg Curl	3. Leg Press
4. Calf Raise	4. Leg Curl
5. Lateral Raise	5. Leg Extension
6. Overhead Press	6. Pullover
7. Pullover	7. Pulldown
8. Arm Cross	8. Decline Press
9. Neck and Shoulder	9. Rowing Torso
10. Triceps Extension	10. Abdominal
11. Biceps Curl	11. Rotary Torso
12. Four-Way Neck	12. Wrist Curl

One set of 8 to 12 repetitions should be performed on each exercise. When 12 or more correct repetitions are performed the resistance should be increased at the next workout.

The largest and strongest muscles of the body are the gluteus maximus of the buttocks. These muscles are being exercised on the Nautilus hip and back machine. (Photo by Art Gutierrez)

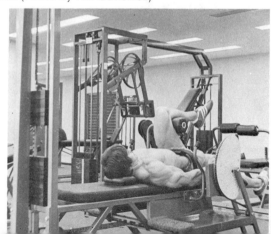

EVERY DAY VS. EVERY OTHER DAY

Q. *On a reducing program, would it help to use Nautilus equipment every day, rather than every other day?*

A. It is important that the dieter train on Nautilus equipment only every other day, or three times a week. The primary objective is not to burn calories but to stimulate the muscles to get stronger. Stronger muscles in turn burn more calories under all resting and working conditions.

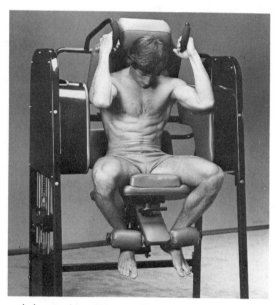

The Nautilus abdominal machine will strengthen and condition the most important muscles of the midsection. But it will not remove large amounts of fatty tissue from the waistline. When fat is lost, it is lost gradually from all over the body and not from one specific area.

ACTIVITY ON NON-NAUTILUS DAYS

Q. *What about doing some type of sporting activity, such as tennis or bicycling, on the non-Nautilus days?*

A. As long as sporting activities are participated in on a low-intensity level, no harm will be done. But any sporting activity can become a demanding activity if the work load is drastically increased. High-intensity activities quickly drain a person's recovery ability. Adequate levels of recovery ability are a necessary requirement for muscular growth. Activities on the non-Nautilus training days should be of a light, easy-going nature.

gaining weight

DESIRE TO GAIN WEIGHT

Q. *How widespread is the desire to gain weight?*

A. A recent Gallup Youth Survey found that among teen-age boys (13 to 18 years old), 35% wanted to gain weight, 33% wanted to lose weight, and 32% were satisfied with their present weight. Among teenage girls, the picture was quite different. Two-thirds of the teenage girls questioned said they would like to lose weight.

The accompanying table shows that the desire to gain weight is primarily a male attitude. This attitude seems to be more prevalent among boys in the older teen group.

Gallup Youth Survey
Do You Want to Gain or Lose Weight?

	Gain	Lose	Stay Same
Nationwide	24%	50%	26%
Boys	35%	33%	32%
13–15 years old	33%	37%	30%
16–18 years old	37%	30%	33%
Girls	14%	65%	21%
13–15 years old	15%	62%	23%
15–18 years old	13%	70%	17%

Note: The survey results are based on a representative sample of 1,012 teenagers from across the nation, interviewed by telephone in October 1979.

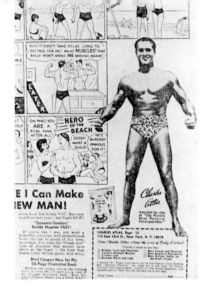

Millions of teenagers have responded to the famous Charles Atlas advertisement, that has remained virtually unchanged for more than 50 years. "Of the 250,000 inquiries we get each year about our mail-order courses," said a company executive, "the majority of the writers are interested in gaining weight—solid weight—in the right places."

FAT AND MUSCLE

Q. *What happens when a person gains weight? Where does the weight go?*

A. Much of this answer depends on what the individual does to promote the weight gain.

The human body can be considered a four-compartmental system:

Body weight = fat + extracellular water + muscle cells + bone minerals.

Of these four, the ones most likely to undergo measurable changes are fat and muscle cells.

Body fat is composed of subcutaneous fat, depot fat, and essential fat. Subcutaneous fat consists of layers of fat found directly under the skin all over the body. It makes up the major percentage of fat in most individuals. Depot fat is usually deposited in the abdominal region in men and around the hips and thighs in women. Essential fat is necessary for the normal maintenance of the body. It makes up the covering of nerves and the membranes of cells and it cushions and protects many vital organs of the body.

There are also three types of muscle in the human body, differing both in structure and function: skeletal, smooth, and cardiac. Skeletal muscles attach to bones and their contractions allow us to move. Smooth muscles are basically involuntary and make up our internal organs. Cardiac or heart muscle is unique in that it has spontaneous contractibility and extremely rapid recovery.

The human body has a tremendous capacity to increase the size of subcutaneous and depot fat cells. Food calories over and above an individual's daily energy requirements lead to a slow but sure increase in body fat (3,500 calories equal a pound of fat).

The body also has a great capacity to increase the size of skeletal muscle cells. While calories are necessary in gaining muscle (600 calories in a pound of muscle), exercise that stimulates the muscles to grow larger and stronger is of far greater importance.

When weight gain occurs in the body (outside the natural maturation process and pregnancy), what is actually happening is an increase in fat or muscle, or both fat and muscle.

GAINING MUSCLE, NOT FAT

Q. *From a fitness point of view, it would be advantageous to gain muscle weight and not fat weight. Is this correct?*

A. Right! Muscle cells are active. Much of their time is spent contracting and stretching. Fat cells, however, are fairly inactive. They do not have much in the way of metabolic activity and can function on considerably less oxygen than muscle cells.

Fat does not contribute to muscular contraction. Fat between muscle fibers acts as a friction brake and can actually impede the normal, relatively frictionless movement of lean muscle fibers during exercise. In the performance of most sports, muscles contribute everything. Fat contributes nothing!

As a result, most athletes would perform much better with a greater percentage of muscle mass and a smaller percentage of body fat. Except for long-distance swimming and sumo wrestling, there are no sports for which additional body fat would be an advantage.

The human body contains 434 skeletal muscles. These muscles are our only means of movement. Without muscles we would be little more than vegetables. Any time an individual increases his muscle mass to body weight ratio, he improves his movement potential.

THREE REQUIREMENTS FOR MUSCLE GROWTH

Q. *How does the body gain muscle weight?*

A. As a muscle grows bigger and stronger, it weighs more. Getting the muscles to grow is the key to gaining productive body weight.

Muscle growth consists of three parts. *One,* growth stimulation must take place within the body itself at the basic cellular level. This is best accomplished through high-intensity exercise. *Two,* the proper nutrients must be available for the stimulated cells. But providing nutrients in excess of what the body requires will do nothing to promote growth of muscle fibers. Muscle stimulation must always precede nutrition. If a

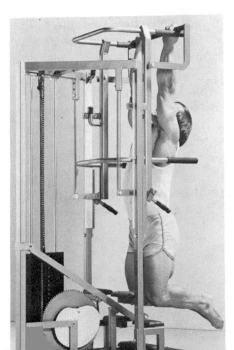

Muscles are stimulated to grow by high-intensity exercise, not by eating certain foods.

person has stimulated muscular growth through high-intensity exercise, his muscles will grow on almost any reasonable diet. *Three,* sufficient time for rest and recovery from strenuous exercise is necessary for muscular growth.

The chemical reactions inside a growing muscle are much more complicated than just exercising, eating, and resting. High-intensity muscular contraction results in the formation of a chemical called creatine. The creatine stimulates the muscle to form more myosin, one of the contraction proteins within the muscle fiber. Myosin impels the muscle to stronger contractions. This results in the production of more creatine.

Creatine is the messenger substance that turns on the ribonucleic acid (RNA) processing line to produce muscle growth. The RNA molecules within a specialized compartment of the cell act as an assembly line and hook together various combinations of amino acids. Sometimes, in combination with complex sugars and fats, the molecules form different compounds that increase the size of certain muscle cells. To gain muscle weight an individual must stimulate growth through high-intensity exercise, then provide rest and the proper nutrients.

UNIMPORTANCE OF PROTEIN

Q. *Why do so many athletes who are trying to build muscle mass consume large amounts of protein foods?*

A. Because they have heard that "muscles are made of protein" and "to build muscle, you need to eat lots of protein." These ideas are simply not true. Only 22% of muscle is protein. More than 70% of muscle is water.

There are about 100 grams of protein, a small amount of fat, a lot of water, and about 600 calories in a pound of muscle. If an athlete stimulated a pound of muscle growth over a week's period of time, he would need to consume an extra 14 grams of protein and 86 calories each day. This is not much in the way of additional food, if any, since the typical athlete probably consumes three times as much protein as he needs per day.

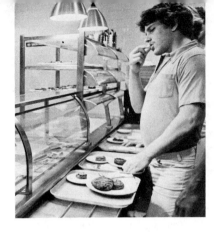

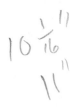

Eating high-protein foods, such as beef-steak, will not stimulate an athlete's muscles to grow. It will, however, stimulate his fat cells to increase in size if his caloric input for the day exceeds his caloric output.

GAINING MUSCLE AND LOSING FAT

Q. *Is it possible for a person to gain muscle weight and lose body fat at the same time?*

A. Yes. In fact, this has been recommended for many years by Nautilus Sports/Medical Industries.

Gaining muscle while losing fat at the same time is accomplished through brief, infrequent, high-intensity exercise to stimulate growth in the major muscle groups combined with a balanced, reduced-calorie diet. The diet, about 500 calories below maintenance level, causes a gradual decrease in body fat. The high-intensity exercise causes a gradual increase in muscle mass. Research with animals has shown that muscular growth can occur in rats fed zero calories, just water, if they were exercised properly beforehand. Evidently, since a pound of fat contains 3,500 calories and a pound of muscle contains only 600 calories, the body can convert fat into the necessary raw materials to produce muscle mass. Of course, the muscles first must be stimulated to grow through high-intensity exercise.

A high-intensity Nautilus program would consist of four to six exercises for the lower body and six to eight exercises for the upper body. One set of 8 to 12 repetitions, with as much weight as possible, should be performed every other day, or three times a week. More resistance should be added when 12 or more repetitions can be executed in correct form.

A SIMPLE TEST

Q. *Other than weight alone, is there a simple way to tell if a person is losing fat and building muscle at the same time?*

A. If a person wants to know how fast he is gaining muscle and losing fat, he can keep a weekly record of the difference between his relaxed and contracted arm measurements. If he is lean and muscular, he will usually have a difference of one to two inches. If he has more than a minimum amount of fat, he will have less than a one-inch difference.

The reason for this contrast between the measurements of a lean person and an overly fat one is, as the physiologists say, "You can't flex fat." Only muscle contains contractile tissue. Since fat is reduced proportionally all over the body and most noncontractile fat is stored around the hips and midsection, a person may have a 1-inch layer of fat over the side of the waist and a $\frac{1}{4}$-inch layer on the back of the arm. When the 1-inch measurement is reduced to $\frac{1}{2}$ inch, the $\frac{1}{4}$-inch measurement will be reduced to $\frac{1}{8}$ inch.

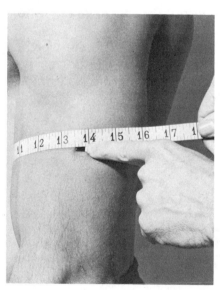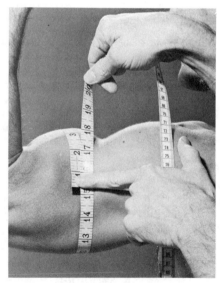

Measure the individual's hanging arm midway between the elbow and the tip of the shoulder. The tape in the first photograph reads 13$\frac{1}{2}$ inches. With the upper arm parallel with the floor and the biceps fully flexed, place the tape at a right angle to the bone. The flexed measurement is 15 inches. The difference between the person's hanging and flexed biceps is 1$\frac{1}{2}$ inches, an indication of a small amount of body fat.

In recording weekly arm measurement, the following rules should be observed:

1. Take the measurements before a training session.

2. Use the same tape measure for every measurement. A cloth sewing tape is best for this purpose.

3. Relax the arm and take the measurement midway between the elbow and the tip of the shoulder with the arm hanging away from the body. Record to the nearest $\frac{1}{16}$ inch.

4. Flex the arm and measure it at right angles to the bone around the largest part of the flexed biceps with the upper arm parallel to the floor. Record this also to the nearest $\frac{1}{16}$ inch.

5. Take the difference between the relaxed and the contracted measurements.

NAUTILUS WORKOUT FOR GAINING MUSCLE WEIGHT

Q. *What is a good Nautilus workout for a teenage boy who wants to gain muscle?*

A. The teenage boy who is trying to gain muscle weight should concentrate on exercising the largest muscles of the body. The following Nautilus exercises should be performed on an every-other-day schedule.

1. Hip & Back
2. Stiff-Legged Deadlift
3. Leg Extension
4. Leg Press
5. Hip Abduction
6. Hip Adduction
7. Pullover
8. Negative Chin
9. Arm Cross
10. Negative Dip
11. Neck & Shoulder

NAUTILUS VS. BARBELLS

Q. *It has been said that Nautilus does not build bulky muscles like barbells do. Is this correct?*

A. Bulky muscles are primarily a result of genetics. In order to have very large or bulky muscles an individual must have long muscle bellies and short tendon attachments. Then he must train these muscles in a high-intensity manner. If a person has the genetic potential to have large muscles, Nautilus will provide much faster results than will training with barbells.

BUILDING BULK FOR FOOTBALL

Q. *How do football players gain bulk?*

A. Gaining bulk to most football players and coaches means getting fatter by eating more calories. Additional fat would make a defensive lineman harder to move, at least from an offensive lineman's point of view. But it also will make the player slower, less coordinated, less healthy, and more prone to heart disease in later life.

Force feeding of football players is the rule at most college training tables because very few coaches and athletes realize that such eating causes much more harm than good.

It is to a football coach's advantage to have his athletes as lean and muscular as possible. He should motivate his athletes to gain muscle, not fat.

The concept of gaining bulk is misleading. What athletes and coaches should strive to increase is skeletal muscle mass and decrease body fat stores. Both of these goals can be accomplished through high-intensity, progressive exercise along with a balanced diet.

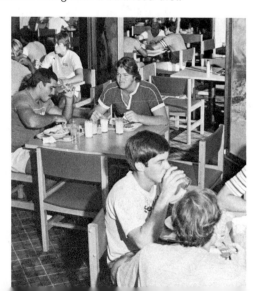

HIGH-CALORIE DIET

Q. *What about the athletes who are actually underfat? Is a high-calorie diet recommended for them?*

A. Many coaches believe they have athletes who are underfat. These athletes are probably undermuscled rather than underfat. Although underfat people do exist in other countries, it would be difficult to find athletes in the United States who are lacking in fat. Occasionally, teenage athletes have high metabolic rates or bodies that are inefficient at utilizing calories. If this is the case, the chart in Chapter 3 can be used in developing a high-calorie diet.

ANOREXIA NERVOSA

Q. *Would a young girl suffering from anorexia nervosa profit from gaining fat?*

A. Yes, but there are many other factors to consider as well.

Anorexia nervosa is a life-threatening disorder of deliberate self-starvation with wide-ranging physical and psychiatric components. The person is obsessed with the idea of not eating food. Because of emotional problems, she denies her hunger and does not eat, or goes on a food binge, then vomits or takes laxatives.

Q. *What kind of people are susceptible to anorexia nervosa?*

A. The illness usually occurs during adolescence and young adulthood as an aftermath of a reducing diet. Most victims are white females from middle- and upper-class families. The parents are usually conscientious, educated, well-meaning people who are high achievers themselves.

Q. *What are the signs and symptoms?*

A. Anorexia nervosa may include:

1. 20–40% body weight loss
2. Cessation of menstrual periods

3. Hyperactivity
4. Distorted body image
5. Food binges followed by fasting, vomiting, or using laxatives
6. Excessive constipation
7. Depression
8. Loss of hair (head)
9. Growth of fine body hair
10. Intolerance to cold temperatures
11. Low pulse rate
12. Lack of subcutaneous fat

Q. *What are the consequences and treatments for anorexia?*

A. Some people will recover completely, some will lead a borderline existence, and some will die.

The best treatment is a combination of medical, nutritional, and psychotherapy for the patient as well as counseling for other family members.

STEROID DRUGS FOR GAINING WEIGHT

Q. *Are steroid drugs an effective way for an athlete to gain weight?*

A. The most popular drugs used at the present time by athletes are androgenic-anabolic steroids. Androgenic refers to the production of masculine characteristics, while anabolic relates to the conversion of food within a cell. These drugs are synthetic forms of testosterone and other male hormones. A few of the most common brands are Dianabol, Winstrol, Anavar, Nilevar, Durabolin, and Methyltestosterone. In males it is presumed that the presence of androgens in increased quantities contributes to greater strength and muscle mass. As a result, athletes, especially the marginal ones, have been consuming the drugs.

From a chemical standpoint, these drugs cannot stimulate muscular growth. They cannot increase muscular strength.

But they can cause a person to retain fluids, which accounts for the gain in bodyweight. They also can cause an individual to think he is stronger. This is basically a result of "placebo power," a well-known phenomenon in medicine.

Although the steroid drugs are real medicines, not inactive substances, what they are able to do and what they are believed to do are worlds apart. Androgenic-anabolic steroids are useful in the treatment of some anemias, osteoporosis of the bone, chronic debilitating illnesses, and male hormone deficiencies. But they do not make a healthy athlete bigger, stronger, or faster.

The fact that the steroid drugs do not work from a chemical point of view would be relatively insignificant if there were not harmful side effects. Recently, a physician at a large New York hospital examined more than 300 athletes who had been consuming large amounts of steroid drugs. He emphatically stated that he could detect clinical damage in 100% of the athletes up to six months after the drugs were discontinued,

The use of anabolic steroids has been banned in amateur sport. Urine tests to detect them were developed in 1973 and are now used in international competitions. Steroid testing, however, is expensive and encourages the idea that athletes may gain an advantage by taking these drugs. The main abusers of steroid drugs today tend to be weight lifters and bodybuilders. (Photo by David Ponsonby)

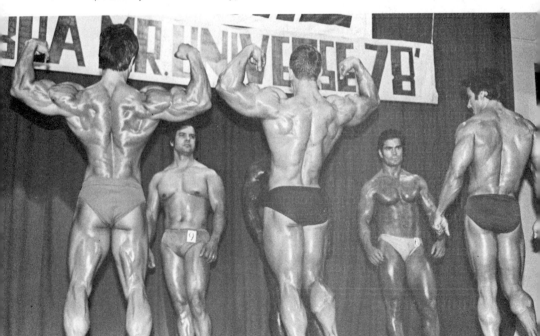

and permanent damage in more than 25% of the athletes. This damage was primarily in the form of one or more of the following: testicular atrophy, pituitary inhibition, prostate hypertrophy, fluid retention (high blood pressure), kidney damage (hardening of the kidney arteries), or impaired liver function (fibrosis).

All athletes using drugs in hopes that they will increase their performance would be wise to remember the following statement from Arthur Jones, owner of Nautilus Sports/Medical Industries:

"There is no known drug that will improve the performance of a healthy athlete . . . and there never will be such a drug; normal health being just that, normal . . . super health, by definition, being impossible."

PLACEBO EFFECT

Q. *What exactly is meant by* placebo power *or* placebo effect?

A. The term *placebo* comes directly from the Latin word meaning "I will please." A standard dictionary definition is "a preparation containing no medicine but given for its psychological effect." Often, the placebo effect is achieved with substances such as sugar pills or injections of sterile water.

The placebo effect, however, includes much more than the use of substances. The term can be used to cover all nonspecific aspects of treatment. For example, the patient's beliefs and expectations, the physician's beliefs and expectations, and the psychological interaction between the two people.

The runner who takes a tablespoon of wheat germ oil before sprinting the fastest 100-meter dash of his life gives the credit to the oil. The bodybuilder who is injected with an anabolic steroid trains harder and notices a gradual increase in the size of his arm. Or the basketball coach who continues to wear the same coat and tie to every game because his team is on a winning streak. Placebo use may have increased their self-confidence.

Q. *If the placebo effect makes someone feel or perform better, what is wrong with that?*

A. The problem is not with the placebo effect itself, but with the people who misunderstand its power and do not give credit where it is due. The athlete who relies on the placebo effect is pretending that he knows what he is doing. The reason he ran the best race of his life was related mostly to his training and maturation, not to the wheat germ oil. An athlete who uses food supplements is encouraging himself to form lifelong habits of using things he does not need.

The majority of people who use placebos do not get positive results. Thus, these practices are not only misleading; they are also a financial rip-off.

Athletes, coaches, and fitness-minded people should base their confidence in sound physiological training methods. The *belief* in sound physiological training methods is the strongest of all placebo effects.

17

focusing on women

TEENAGE GIRLS AND NUTRITION

Q. *Are there reasons why teenage girls are less well nourished than boys?*

A. Yes there are. Teenage girls need almost as much protein, vitamins, and minerals as do teenage boys. But they require, and usually wish to eat, only two-thirds to three-fourths of the quantity of food eaten by boys. To eat well, they must choose more carefully. Also, menstruation increases their need for protein and iron. One *cultural* reason for poor diets among teeange girls is a concern with overweight, based on an unrealistic ideal of what their figures ought to be like. A teenage girl who can model fashions may be a nutritional question mark.

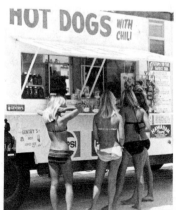

To remain lean and still be well-nourished, teenage girls should choose their foods wisely. (Photo by Ellington Darden)

287

EATING HABITS AND PERFORMANCE

Q. *What habits should a coach encourage to derive the best physical performances from teenage girl athletes?*

A. If teenage athletes are eager eaters, the coach worries that they are eating the wrong things. If they are meager eaters, the coach worries about malnutrition. Either way, inconsistent eating habits could affect their performances on the athletic field. Unfortunately, he could be right!

The coach can do his part by challenging each of his athletes to assume personal responsibility for a year-round schedule of regular exercise, sleep, and well-balanced meals.

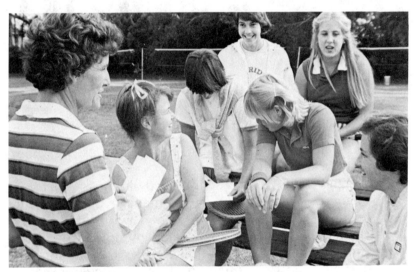

One of the responsibilities of a coach is to see that her girls eat a nutritious breakfast. A nutritious breakfast should include at least 25 percent of the recommended dietary allowance of each essential nutrient.

He should encourage teenage girls to eat more vegetables, especially the green leafy ones, as they are usually neglected. And he should insist that the athletes eat breakfast.

IMPORTANCE OF BREAKFAST

Q. *Why is breakfast such an important meal?*

A. Studies have shown that many teenage girls are listless and inattentive during morning class hours because of poor breakfasts. In one study, of those girls who had poor breakfasts, only one in five ended the day with an adequate diet.

If left to their own devices to choose breakfast food, girls tend to choose poorly, according to a University of California study. Coaches should help the girls learn to like breakfast by encouraging them to eat a wide variety of foods.

Examples of nutritious breakfasts are as follows:

1. ¼ cantaloupe
2. 2 ounces tuna fish
3. 2 slices toast with margarine
4. 1 glass skimmed milk

1. Fresh orange or grapefruit sections
2. Peanut butter and banana sandwich
3. 1 scrambled egg
4. 1 glass skimmed milk

FOOD SUPPLEMENTS AND FEMALE ATHLETES

Q. *Should vitamins and other food supplements be routinely given to female athletes?*

A. No! A balanced diet made up of the previously described Basic Four Food Groups will provide all the nutrients needed by most athletes.

If taking vitamin pills would truly make the difference between winning and losing, tennis champion Billie Jean King would have never been able to defeat Bobby Riggs. Riggs was taking 300 to 400 nutrient pills a day in preparation for the so-called "Battle of the Sexes," or "Tennis Match of the Century." His advisor, Rheo H. Blair, a Hollywood health food advocate and pseudonutritionist, was certain Riggs would be unbeatable after this *supercharged, pill-popping program* had

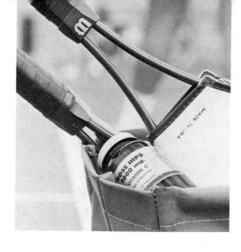

Vitamin pills do not provide pep and energy. Neither are vitamins cure-alls for fatigue and tiredness.

been initiated. The millions of Americans who followed the match should now know better. Such overloads of nutrients are certainly not needed and can lead to dangerous complications.

For example, there is a case of a four-year-old boy in Kansas who took a whole bottle of 40 children's vitamin pills at once. He spent the following two days in intensive care with vitamin A and iron poisoning. His experience was added to the statistics compiled by the National Clearinghouse for Poison Control Centers, which reveal that 4,000 cases of vitamin poisoning are reported each year.

IMPORTANCE OF IRON

Q. *Nutritionists say many women are deficient in iron. Should iron pills be available to women athletes?*

A. Many women are deficient in iron. An athlete who shows signs of unusual fatigue at about midseason should be sent to a physician to have her hemoglobin checked. If the iron in her blood is low, the physician will prescribe the appropriate iron supplement.

The body can absorb only about one-tenth of the iron consumed. Females, therefore, need about 18 milligrams of iron a day to extract the 1 to 2 milligrams needed. Good sources of iron are meats, enriched breads and cereal, leafy vegetables, and dried fruits. Dried apricots and raisins are excellent iron-rich snacks for athletes. They should wash

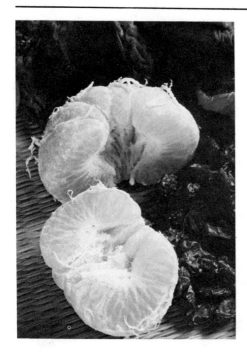

Foods containing 25 milligrams of vitamin C can more than double the amount of iron absorbed from iron-rich foods eaten at the same meal.

them down with orange juice because vitamin C is helpful in the intestinal tract for the absorption of iron.

Normal menstruation involves a small loss of iron and protein, both of which will easily be replaced by good nutrition throughout the month. Approximately 5% of female athletes will have excessive menstrual flows. Those in this group should be sure to increase their consumption of iron-rich foods, especially before and during their periods.

ORAL CONTRACEPTIVE PILLS

Q. *Do women taking oral contraceptive pills have special nutritional needs?*

A. Women using oral contraceptives may need more vitamin B_6, B_{12}, folic acid, A, and C, perhaps because their bodies may handle them differently.

Research also shows that the need for iron and copper may be decreased by oral contraceptives. These two minerals are essential for the formation of hemoglobin, the oxygen-carrying pigment of the red blood cells. In addition, a woman's menstrual flow is often lighter on oral contraceptives, so iron losses decrease. This is good news, since the Recommended Dietary Allowances for iron, 18 milligrams, is difficult for many women to meet from diet alone.

In practical terms, what does this mean to a woman who is on oral contraceptive pills? She should make certain that she eats a varied, balanced diet. In particular, she should include good sources of the B vitamins, A, and C. Excellent sources include meats, particularly liver, fish, and poultry; dairy products; enriched and whole-grain breads; potatoes and other vegetables, especially dark yellow and leafy green ones; citrus fruits, tomatoes, and melons.

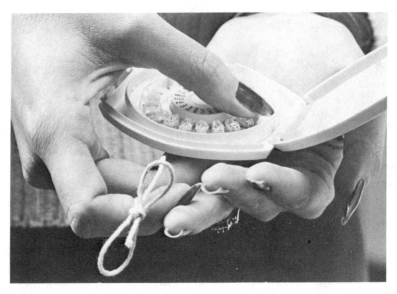

Oral contraceptive drugs increase blood levels of some nutrients and decrease blood levels of others. A woman taking these pills should remember to consume foods rich in vitamins A, B, and C.

WEIGHT GAIN DURING PREGNANCY

Q. *What is the proper amount of weight a woman should gain during pregnancy?*

A. A normal and desirable weight to gain during the nine months of pregnancy is about 24 pounds. During the first trimester only a small weight gain is noted, usually 3 pounds. Approximately 9 pounds are gained during the second trimester and an additional 12 pounds during the third trimester.

The following chart details the specifics of the weight gain during pregnancy:

Development	Weight Gain (pounds)
Infant at birth	7½
Placenta	1
Increase in mother's blood volume to supply placenta	4
Increase in size of mother's uterus and muscles to support it	2½
Increase in size of mother's breasts	3
Fluid to surround infant in amniotic sac	2
Mother's fat stores	4
Total	24 pounds

NUTRITIONAL REQUIREMENTS DURING PREGNANCY

Q. *Are there additional nutrition requirements of a pregnant woman?*

A. During pregnancy the need for most nutrients can be said to rise about 30% above normal during the second trimester and climb to about 50% above normal during the last three months. For the first three months of pregnancy, food needs do not change from those of a normal balanced diet.

Calorie needs *do not increase*—except during the last trimester. Even then the caloric requirements of a pregnant woman go up only about 10%. Any calories beyond this increase are likely to make fat mothers and fat babies. The overfat baby does not have as good a chance for normal birth and survival. The mother who becomes fat during pregnancy has a strong tendency to retain that fat.

Pregnancy is a state that should be kept under medical supervision, and dietary management is an important part of that supervision. Obstetricians have long taken careful note of research into the effects of food on pregnancy and lactation. The qualified specialist in obstetrics is a woman's best dietary consultant during pregnancy.

Though most nutritionists feel that nearly all the dietary needs of pregnancy can easily be met by a sound diet, most obstetricians play it safe by prescribing some vitamin and mineral supplements once pregnancy is diagnosed. The pregnant woman is warned not to follow the "more is better" philosophy with food or supplements or the idea of "eating for two." The woman who does so risks her welfare and that of the baby.

The nutritive needs during pregnancy are best met by a wholesome diet, the basis of which is milk, cheese, meat, eggs, nuts, legumes, grains, vegetables, especially dark green, leafy ones, and fruits.

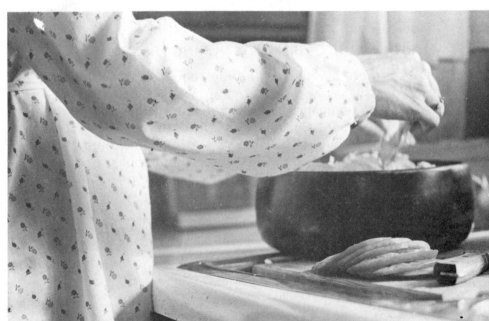

Q. *Are there any other things not to do from a nutritional point of view during pregnancy?*

A. Yes, several facts should be brought to a pregnant woman's attention:

1. *Do not drink alcoholic beverages.* Alcohol quickly enters not only the bloodstream of the mother but also that of the fetus. This means that the fetus can become drunk and suffer other ills from the alcohol. Furthermore, many babies born to women who drink during pregnancy have alcohol fetal syndrome, a condition characterized by low birth weight, slowed growth and development, and sometimes permanent mental retardation.

2. *Do not smoke.* Smoking during pregnancy decreases infant birth weight. The more a mother smokes, the greater the effects. In addition, women who smoke are much more likely to suffer miscarriages than nonsmokers. Those who cannot quit smoking completely should at least cut back as much as possible.

3. *Do not go on reducing diets.* Pregnancy is not the time for a woman to reduce calories in an attempt to lose body fat. It is certainly a time, however, when she needs to be particularly conscious of selecting foods with high-nutrient density. In general, the more fruits and vegetables eaten the better, because these foods help to ensure a sufficiency of vitamins and minerals without appreciably increasing caloric intake.

4. *Do not consume products that are high in caffeine.* Noting that caffeine is a stimulant with a definite drug effect, the Federal Drug Administration recently recommended that pregnant women avoid products containing caffeine or to use them sparingly. Coffee, tea, and cola drinks are the most widely consumed foods that contain appreciable amounts of caffeine.

NUTRITIONAL REQUIREMENTS OF NURSING MOTHERS

Q. *Does the nursing mother need the same amount of food as she required while pregnant?*

A. The nursing mother needs more food than she required during pregnancy. Once nursing is established, she often produces more than a quart of milk a day. She needs more protein, vitamins, calcium, and other minerals. All these nutrients can be attained by eating the same wholesome foods she ate during pregnancy—only in greater quantities. The woman's obstetrician should manage her diet during pregnancy as well as in nursing.

BREAST-FEEDING

Q. *Is breast milk still the best food for the infant?*
A. Yes! The milk of a human mother is much better designed for the infant than is the milk of a cow. Mother's milk provides immunities against disease whereas formulas made with cow's milk do not. Furthermore, mother's milk does not ordinarily cause infant digestive upsets. Another advantage of breast-feeding is that the nervous stimulation of the breast by the baby's sucking causes the release of hormones within the mother's body that accelerate the return of the uterus to its normal size.

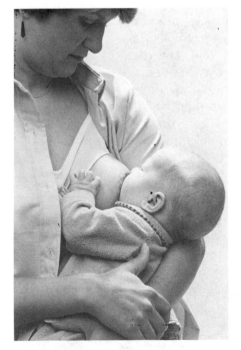

For a nursing mother, diet is of extra importance because she is nourishing the child through her own body.

A woman who cannot breast-feed, however, should be assured that science is now able to provide excellent nutrition for the bottle-fed baby.

EXERCISE DURING PREGNANCY

Q. *Will a regular exercise program make childbirth easier?*

A. To answer this question with a *yes* requires nothing more than common sense, according to Dr. Clayton Thomas. "If you could separate all the people on earth into those who exercise and those who do not, who do you think would be the healthiest and have the easiest time having babies? It would be a paradox if the sedentary person had fewer problems. I know of no evidence that exercise is harmful in a normal pregnancy.

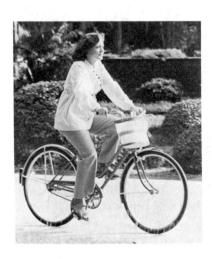

Women who remain active during pregnancy have greater flexibility in their food choices than do women who are inactive.

Q. *Should a woman athlete discontinue competition during pregnancy?*

A. Noticeable changes in athletic performance first show up at the end of the third month. Most mothers gain only about three pounds during the first trimester, but during the second trimester the uterus expands 20 times and a woman will gain about nine pounds. This extra weight, a protruding abdomen, a loss of balance, and the effects of water retention and anemia may simply make sports competition too complicated. Even the well-trained athlete will find it difficult to do her best at this point.

Because of this deterioration in performance, most athletes give up competition but not exercise by the third month. A woman who is used to competition and heavy training could safely compete beyond this time. Physicians get a bit alarmed when they hear of these efforts and recommend that athletes stop competition by the sixth month of pregnancy. But there is no scientific evidence that competition during pregnancy is harmful, and a woman should judge when it is time to quit by the way she feels.

MISCARRIAGE DEFINED

Q. *Exactly what is miscarriage? Is there danger of miscarriage if a woman competes in vigorous sport?*

A. A miscarriage means that the fetus is born before it is capable of surviving outside the mother's body. The majority of miscarriages occur during the second or third month of pregnancy while a small number occur as late as the seventh month. Microscopic examinations of miscarried embryos and fetuses reveal that more than 80% of them have biological deformity that would make them unable to survive and live a normal life. A miscarriage, in most instances, should be considered one of nature's own built-in controls. Any unusual bleeding from the vagina, however, should be reported to a physician.

There is very little danger of miscarriage from vigorous sport participation, especially if the woman is accustomed to the activity. The fetus is well-cushioned. It floats in a sack of fluid that works like a shock absorber. A pregnant woman cannot jiggle a baby loose by running, jumping, or horseback riding. Nor can she harm it by swimming. Very strong stomach blows or falls in the eighth or ninth month might start labor contractions prematurely. Physicians, therefore, advise against vigorous or contact sports toward the end of pregnancy.

STRETCH MARKS

Q. *Does every pregnant woman get stretch marks? How can they be prevented?*

A. Stretch marks are caused by the tearing of the elastic tissues in the skin that is associated with enlargement of breasts, distention of the abdomen, or the deposition of subcutaneous fat. Stretch marks appear as pink or purplish-red lines during pregnancy. The lines become permanent grayish-white scarlike marks after delivery. Some women never develop stretch marks despite bearing several children. Others lose most of the tone in their skin after one pregnancy. Evidently there is an inherited factor involved in stretch marks.

Stretch marks cannot be considered evidence that a woman has borne a child, however, because they sometimes are seen in women who have never been pregnant.

Once a woman gets stretch marks, there is nothing she can do about them. She might help to prevent them by making sure she does not gain excessive amounts of body fat.

VARICOSE VEINS

Q. *How are varicose veins related to pregnancy?*

A. Varicose veins can be seen as bulging, twisted, and knotted veins that are usually located right under the skin. While they frequently occur in pregnant women, they also appear in other women and men as well. Most often they develop in the legs, although they can pop out in other places. When they appear in the anal area, they are called hemorrhoids. Their presence is due to two factors: One, many pregnancies contribute to a generally weakened condition of the veins in the legs if the pressure created by the baby cuts off some circulation. Two, varicose veins can be inherited. In such a case, the individual probably has a tendency toward inelasticity in the walls of the veins.

In both instances, however, the results are the same: there is a weakness or malfunction within the flaplike valves of the vein. As the pressure of the blood on the vein increases, the vein bulges. After continuous stretching it loses its elasticity.

Q. *Will exercise help varicose veins?*

A. Yes. Any type of contracting or pumping of the leg muscles helps to milk the blood out of the calves and thighs and propel it upward toward the heart. Brisk walking is good exercise. Calf raises and squats are even better. All women can benefit by maintaining muscle tone in the thigh and calf muscles. The strong, firm muscles around the deep veins help provide external support and help protect them from overstretching and damage.

NAUTILUS FOR WOMEN

Q. *Does Nautilus exercise make a woman develop large muscles?*

A. Most women believe that, if they do heavy exercises, their muscles will become large and unfeminine. But it is virtually impossible for a woman to develop large muscles.

Building large muscles requires two factors. First, the individual must have long muscle bellies and short tendon attachments. Second, an adequate amount of male hormones, particularly testosterone, must be present in the bloodstream. Women almost never have either of these factors.

Under no circumstances could 99.99% of American women develop large muscles. Nautilus exercise is important for them because it can strengthen muscles, prevent injuries, and turn the body into trimmer and more shapely flesh.

Q. *What about all those women Olympic athletes with large muscles?*

A. The vast majority of women involved in Olympic and

professional sports have slim, well-toned bodies. It is unfortunate that certain photographs and publicity have led people to believe that women athletes with large muscles are the rule rather than the rare exception.

During the Moscow Olympic Games, there were many very tall women playing basketball. One Russian player, Iuli Semenova, was 7 feet 2 inches tall. A teammate of hers measured 6 feet 8 inches tall. Most of the women on the medal-winning teams were over 6 feet tall.

Suppose that, after watching several Olympic basketball games, a woman wondered whether bouncing a ball would make her taller. She might try various ball-bouncing routines with no success and conclude that bouncing a ball had no effect on increasing her height. She might then realize that, if she grew in height, it would be due to her genetic inheritance and not her ball bouncing.

This is the case for the very few women with large muscles. They have inherited above-average length to their muscles and above-average levels of male hormones. They have the ability to develop larger and more defined muscles than the typical woman. These few women will be larger and stronger than the average woman even if they never exercise or take part in sports.

If a woman who had all the genetic capabilities actually did develop unsightly muscles, she could go without exercise for a week and her muscles would shrink. Muscles are made to be used. If they are not used, they atrophy.

SPOT REDUCING

Q. *Are there Nautilus exercises that will assist a woman in spot reducing fatty deposits on her hips?*

A. Spot reducing is not possible. Many people, however, believe that concentrated exercise for a body part that is laden with fat will be effective in removing the fat. Although exercise does play a role in reduction of body fat when combined with proper diet, the fat is mobilized out of fat cells all over the body.

Where a woman stores and loses fat is inherited. Try as she may, she cannot change her patterns of fat distribution. This does not mean that proper Nautilus exercise will not benefit her. The hip and leg machines will strengthen the muscles of the lower body, and the fat and skin that surround these muscles will become somewhat tighter and firmer.

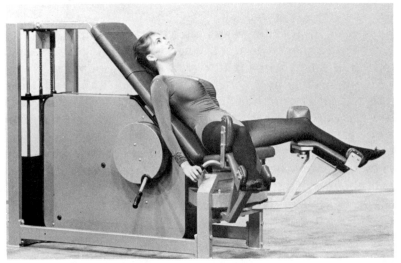

The hip abduction movement performed on the Nautilus hip abduction/ adduction machine will firm and tighten the muscles of the outer hips. (Photo by Inge Cook)

FAT LOSS AND BREAST SHAPE

Q. *What can be done to prevent breast shrinkage during a fat-reduction program?*
A. The breasts are largely made up of fat and possess no voluntary muscle. Since a fat-loss program burns fat throughout the body, the breasts may also become smaller. Breast shape and contour, however, will improve if the supporting muscular layer beneath them is properly strengthened. The Nautilus double chest and pullover machines offer full-range exercise for these muscles.

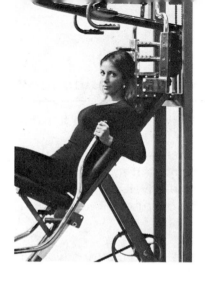

The Nautilus double chest machine is specifically designed to strengthen and shape the large muscles that underlie the breasts. (Photo by Inge Cook)

EMOTIONAL PROBLEMS

Q. *Can emotional problems contribute to an overfat condition?*

A. Yes. These problems may range from occasional nervous tension to deep-seated disturbances. Lean people tend to eat less when they are under tension while their fatter peers tend to stuff themselves.

GLANDULAR PROBLEMS

Q. *If a glandular problem is diagnosed in a woman, is it possible that this will contribute to her overfat condition?*

A. The secretions of different glands in the body can affect growth, even fatty growth. A malfunction of these sensitive organs may result in a tendency for a woman to be fat, but she must realize that the resulting fat stores cannot be accumulated without calorie-containing foodstuff. For details on glandular conditions, consult a physician.

DIURETICS AND WATER RETENTION

Q. *Are diuretics useful in a fat-loss program?*

A. The use of diuretics as a part of a woman's fat-loss program is strongly discouraged. Diuretics are chemical substances that rid the body of excessive water. A woman must remember, however, that there is very little water in fat. The weight loss from diuretics is not from fatty deposits.

Women who self-administer diuretics may deplete their stores of potassium and other substances. If too much potassium is lost, blood pressure may drop adversely, and serious problems can occur. In addition, the overuse of diuretics can irritate the kidneys or raise blood sugar.

Q. *Why does body weight suddenly plateau after a woman has faithfully followed her reduction program for a week or so?*

A. Certain women tend to retain fluid as they lose fat. Even though they are losing fat, it does not show on the scale, at least not for several weeks. This plateau is usually a temporary phenomenon, and after a few weeks, these women will once again begin to lose weight on a low-calorie diet.

The chart on the next page shows the body weight records of Carlene Merry, who was on a 1,200-calorie-a-day diet. It was calculated that she would lose approximately 1½ pounds per week. Many women dieters, as Carlene's chart dramatically reveals, experience a temporary body weight plateau after several weeks. This plateau results not because they are cheating on their diet, but because they have gained water weight temporarily while they are still losing fat. The fat a dieter hopes to lose must be combined with oxygen (oxidized) to make carbon dioxide and water if it is to leave the body. The oxygen she inhales combines with the carbons of the fat to make carbon dioxide and with the hydrogens to make water. The carbon dioxide will be exhaled quickly. But the water stays in the body for a longer time The water takes a while to leave the cell, then enters the spaces between the cells, then works its way into the lymph system, and finally enters the bloodstream. Only after the water arrives in the blood will the kidneys send it to the bladder for excretion. While water is making its way into the blood, the dieter will have a weight gain, because the water weighs more than the fat that was oxidized. But if a person faithfully follows her low-calorie diet plan, one day the plateau will break. The dieter will know it by her frequent urination.

THE PLATEAU EFFECT

Actual Weight Loss
Calculated Weight Loss

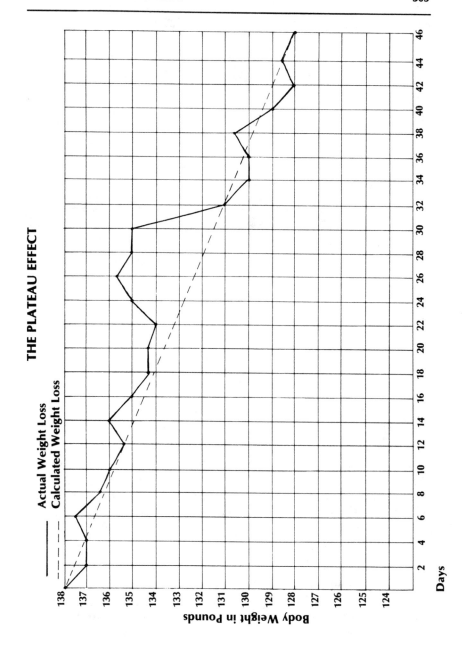

Body Weight in Pounds

Days

putting facts into practice

NUTRIENT NEEDS OF ATHLETES

Q. *Surely it is true that the athlete requires many more, if not different, nutrients than the nonathlete, right?*

A. More than fifty nutrients are required for the building, upkeep, and repair of the human body. With four possible exceptions—calories, water, sodium, and chloride—both the athlete and nonathlete have similar nutritional requirements. Both the athlete and nonathlete, therefore, should try to consume a mixed diet composed of a wide variety of foods.

The biggest difference in nutrient requirements between the athlete and the nonathlete concerns energy, especially during training or conditioning. The amount of energy expended by the athlete during hard training depends on the intensity and duration of the workout as well as the individual's physiological condition and the efficiency or skill of performance. In other words, the novice and unconditioned

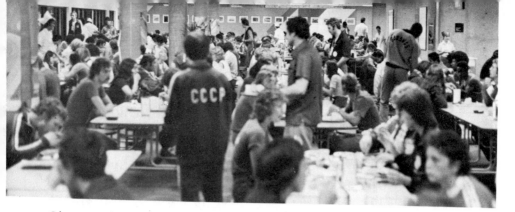

Olympic athletes, in comparison to average people, are unique in that they have inherited the physical potential to excel in a given sport. Olympic athletes, however, are *not* unique in their nutritional requirements. Both athletes and nonathletes require balanced nutrition. (Photo by Ellington Darden)

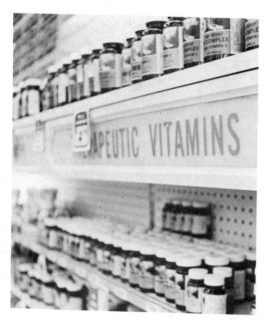

Vitamins are essential to good health. But it is not necessary for a person to obtain vitamins from pills. A balanced diet supplies adequate amounts of all vitamins.

athlete will utilize more energy in playing a game of football or tennis than the skilled and conditioned athlete. Furthermore, those who participate in endurance-type activities expend the most energy. The most efficient and desirable source of energy for these activities is carbohydrate foods.

The other three nutrients, water and sodium chloride (salt), are also more important to the athlete than the nonathlete. These nutrients would be especially important during vigorous training or activity carried out in a hot and humid environment. The athlete must ingest additional water and salt to replenish the losses that occur during these periods of profuse sweating.

ADDITIONAL NUTRITION INFORMATION

Q. *Where can an athlete get sound information on the subjects of food and nutrition?*

A. Generally speaking, the place to go for authoritative information is not another athlete, not the health food stores, and not the library. Libraries try to carry every book published, especially if it is popular, and do not attempt to exercise judgment on its reliability.

This book provides some background material on nutrition as well as the answers to many of the questions athletes and coaches are asking. If additional questions or problems arise, an athlete should consult local or national sources that can provide authoritative information on nutrition and food. Many of the reliable sources provide printed materials, films, exhibits, and consulting or other specialty services. A list of some of these sources follows:

Government Agencies

Food and Drug Administration
Department of Health and Human Services
5600 Fishers Lane
Rockville, MD 20852

National Academy of Science
Food and Nutrition Board
2101 Constitution Ave.
Washington, DC 20418

Department of Agriculture
Publication Inquiry Branch
Washington, DC 20250

Superintendent of Documents
Government Printing Office
Washington, DC 20402

Also, state and local health departments

National Professional Organizations

American Medical Association
535 N. Dearborn St.
Chicago, IL 60610

American Dietetic Association
430 N. Michigan Ave.
Chicago, IL 60601

American Home Economics Association
2010 Massachusetts Ave. NW
Washington, DC 20036

Society for Nutrition Education
2140 Shattuck Ave., Suite 1110
Berkeley, CA 94704

Nutrition Foundation
Office of Education and Public Affairs
888 Seventeenth, NW
Washington, DC 20006

APPROVED DIET BOOKS

Q. *Since there are so many fad books on the market concerning nutrition, health, and dieting, is it possible to get an approved list?*

A. A comprehensive list is available from the Chicago Nutrition Association, 8158 South Kedzie Avenue, Chicago, Illinois 60652, $2. This reference list identifies the authors and categorizes the books as (1) recommended, (2) recommended for special purposes, and (3) not recommended. Most of the references are accompanied by an abstract of the book review that appeared in a nutrition, public health, or medical journal. Although a recently published book may not appear on the list, the author may have written other books of a similar nature that have been reviewed. In this case, the reliability of the latter books could be assumed to be very similar to the earlier books.

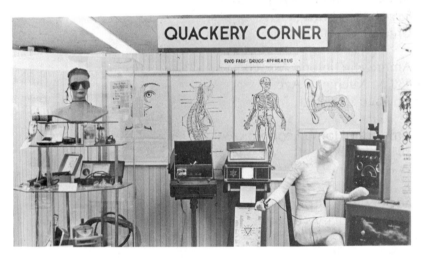

Health Quackery is so prevalent in the United States that it even has a museum all to itself in St. Louis. This photograph shows some of the health frauds that are on display at the National Museum of Medical Quackery. (Photo by Ellington Darden)

SCREENING TESTS

Q. *Are there certain screening tests an individual should get from his personal physician before beginning a reducing diet and Nautilus exercise program?*

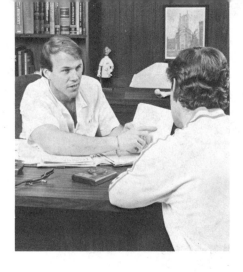

An individual should check with his personal physician before beginning an intensive exercise program or a low-calorie diet. Here, Dr. Michael Fulton, orthopedic surgeon for Nautilus Sports/Medical Industries, gives some exercise guidelines to a patient.

A. Yes, it is always a good idea to check with a physician before beginning a diet and exercise program. The doctor may want to perform some of the following screening tests:

1. Measurement of serum cholesterol and triglycerides
2. Hematocrit
3. Determination of serum uric-acid levels
4. Complete urine analysis
5. Thyroid function tests such as T-3 and T-4
6. Measurement of two-hour postprandial glucose
7. Spirometry or breathing test
8. Chest X ray
9. Resting EKG
10. Stress test EKG that includes blood pressure

BODY WEIGHT MAINTENANCE PROGRAM

Q. *What type of diet should a person adhere to once he has lost his excess body fat?*

A. After losing excess body fat, an individual should be thoroughly familiar with the Basic Four Food Groups: milk, meat, bread and cereal, and fruits and vegetables. Each time a person has a meal he should try to select one small serving of food from each of these groups. Additional foods from the "other foods" group can help add more calories to meals.

A good maintenance program for most women should contain about 1,600 to 1,800 calories a day. Men will need

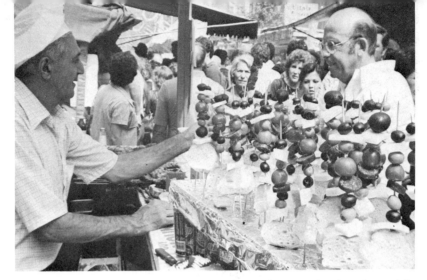

Foods from the Basic Four Food Groups are appetizingly placed on sticks in this photograph. The Basic Four classification is still the single best guideline for fitness-minded people to follow.

slightly more. A person can plan 1,800-calorie menus by simply adding seconds or snacks to the basic 1,200-calorie diet described on page 262. Or he can plan higher-calorie main dishes and desserts that are ordinarily limited.

MODIFIED BASIC FOUR

Q. *Can the Basic Four Food Guide be modified to meet the needs of people who choose not to consume meat or milk?*

A. Yes. Exclusion of meat calls for increases in legumes, nuts, and milk products. If milk and milk products are excluded, more dark green leafy vegetables are needed as a source of calcium. The following table summarizes these recommendations:

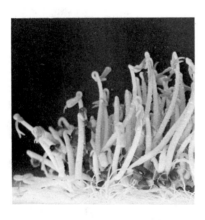

Mung bean sprouts are a rich source of protein, vitamin C, and many B vitamins. They should be consumed when the shoot is between two and three inches long.

Modified Basic Four Food Guides
for Special Preferences

Food Group	No Meat	No Milk
Milk and milk products	4	0
Protein		
Animal sources	0	4
Legumes	2	2
Nuts	1	0
Fruits and vegetables		
Vitamin C-rich	3	3
Dark green	1½	3
Other	3	0
Bread and cereals	6	3

MAKING WEIGHT IN SPORTS

Q. *In sports such as wrestling, judo, and weight lifting, some athletes frequently lose 10 to 15 pounds in a short*

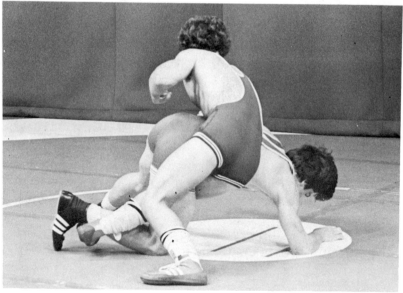

Wrestlers who lose several pounds of body weight the day before an important competition should realize that most of the weight comes from their lean body mass, not their fat stores. (Photo by Inge Cook)

period of time to compete in a lower body weight class. Is this healthy?

A. "Making weight," as this is called, is often accomplished by undergoing very abnormal dietary practices such as starvation and dehydration in order to enter a lower body weight classification. Even though weight classifications are intended to provide an equitable basis for competition, "making weight" allows an athlete to compete against contestants who are normally lighter than he is. This situation is not only unethical but it is also unhealthy and has been condemned by the American Medical Association. There is no healthy, safe way to lose weight fast. And besides, the weight lost in this manner comes mainly from the lean body mass, not from the fat stores.

MUSCLES TURNING TO FAT

Q. *What happens if an athlete exercises and gets into good condition and then stops working out? Will his muscles turn to fat?*

A. Absolutely not! Muscles are muscles, and fat is fat. There is no way an athlete can turn one into the other.

Muscles are composed of 70% water, 22% proteins, and 7% lipids. Fat is 22% water, 6% protein, and 72% lipids. So, like apples and oranges, muscle and fat, though similar in composition, are genetically and chemically different.

When an athlete stops training, he seldom decreases his caloric intake. As a result, he has a gradual decrease in the shape and strength of his muscle mass and an increase in body fat stores. Since muscle and fat are so close to each other that they can intermingle, it appears that his muscles have turned to fat. Fortunately, this does not happen immediately. He can stop exercising completely and work back to his previous level of condition in a fraction of the time it took in the beginning.

NAUTILUS AND FLEXIBILITY

Q. *Will Nautilus exercise make an athlete tight and inflexible?*

A. No. The exact opposite is true. Nautilus exercise, properly performed, will make an athlete more flexible.

Body flexibility is the ability to stretch and contract muscles throughout a full range of motion. The use-or-lose-it principle applies nowhere as cogently as here. Some of the range of motion of a particular muscle can actually be lost if it is not used throughout its full stretching and contracting process. An individual can become tight and inflexible by using his muscles too little—not too much. This can easily be observed in the stiff walk or shuffle of the elderly.

Nautilus exercise applies resistance to the muscles as they are stretched and contracted. Muscles that have been trained in this manner are not only stronger but more flexible.

CALORIES COUNT

Q. *Which is more fattening: one high-calorie dessert or the same caloric consumption spread out over a whole day in a number of servings?*

A. A calorie is a unit of heat energy. It is the only common denominator for measuring the energy value of fats, proteins, and carbohydrates. During any twenty-four hour period, a calorie equals another calorie regardless of its source and when it is consumed.

Many Americans are overfat not because they are snacking between meals but because they are doing exactly what they were trained to do at home. They are eating several well-balanced meals with second helpings each day and cleaning their plates for the starving children in India.

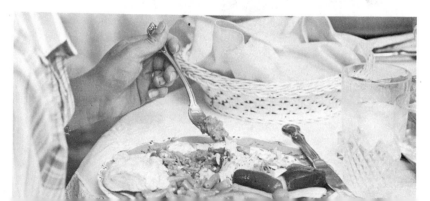

Q. *How can a person count calories when eating out?*

A. Even when eating out, dieters must count calories. This becomes a little more difficult than the food measurements that can be performed at home. After a dieter acquires some experience at home, however, he will quickly learn to estimate food quantities and their caloric values. This is an indispensable asset when eating out.

Q. *In relation to losing fat, does the time of day affect the amount of food eaten?*

A. It is the total number of calories in a several-day period that primarily determines fat loss, not the time of day, the composition of the food, or the amount.

"SLIMMING" FOODS

Q. *Wouldn't an obese person be wise to try to eat more foods that burn themselves up or that do not turn into fat?*

A. Contrary to widespread promotions and promises, there are no such foods. For example, some people think that grapefruit, pineapple, or papaya contain enzymes that myste-

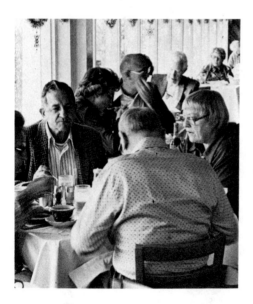

A person who carefully examines a restaurant menu can select a variety of low-calorie foods to meet nutrient needs while losing weight.

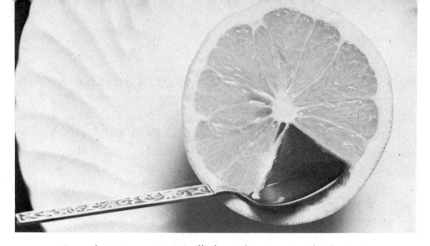
Grapefruit cannot magically burn fat away inside the body.

riously burn up body fat. This is not true. Others commonly believe that protein, unlike other energy sources in our food, is not converted to fat. This, too, is completely false.

All nutrients that provide energy contribute to the total energy pool of the food a person consumes. If the total he takes in is more than he uses, fat is formed.

The body is indifferent to the source of that energy—much as a fireplace does not care whether the heat of its fire comes from pine or oak. But, just as different woods supply different amounts of heat, so do different nutrients supply varying amounts of energy. Protein and carbohydrate each furnish four calories per gram. Fats provide nine calories per gram.

FOOD LEFT IN CANS

Q. *Is it dangerous to leave food in a can that has been opened?*

A. It is safe to keep the food in the original can after it has been opened. The can should be covered and refrigerated, however. A few acid foods may dissolve a little iron from the can, but this is not harmful or dangerous to health. It may cause discoloration of the food product.

FOOD POISONING

Q. *What is food poisoning and how is it caused?*

A. Food poisoning can result from the contamination or

spoilage of food. There are many kinds of food poisoning, and symptoms range from nausea to death. Most commonly, food poisoning is caused by harmful bacteria that are allowed to grow in food and thus produce large quantities of either bacteria or toxin. The most common of these bacteria are salmonella, staphylococcus aureus, and clostridium.

Salmonella enters the body through food, especially raw meats, meat products, eggs, poultry, fish, mayonnaise, milk products, custard, and cream-filled products. Within the digestive tract, salmonella produces a toxin that is damaging to the intestinal cells. After eight to forty-eight hours, the person will experience nausea, vomiting, cramps, diarrhea, chills, and possibly fever.

Staphylococcus aureus is commonly referred to as *staph*. It grows in human nasal passages and infected wounds. Thus, staph is passed on to food by way of people's bodies. Cooks and food handlers are often culprits. Once staph is on a food, it grows best at room temperature and soon a toxin is produced. This toxin cannot be destroyed by cooking. Staph causes disease symptoms similar to salmonella, but they are more severe and occur much sooner, about one to six hours after the toxin-containing food is eaten.

Clostridium represents two kinds of bacteria that cause food-borne diseases: clostridium botulinum and clostridium perfringens.

Clostridium botulinum causes botulism, the most dangerous of all food poisoning. It grows only in the absence of oxygen, such as in vacuum-packed canned goods. An odorless gas and a potent toxin are produced inside the contaminated can. Consuming food from such a can causes flu-like symptoms within twelve to thirty-six hours. It can lead to double vision, dizziness, breathing and swallowing and speech difficulties, and often death. People should be careful to use proper home-canning procedures and not buy or consume foods from cans that have bulges.

Clostridium perfringens is a bacteria that is widespread in nature. It is found in dust, in soil, and in the intestinal tracts of humans and many warm-blooded animals. Clostridium per-fringens grows best in large quantities of foods, especially meats and gravies, that are held at improper temperatures for long periods of time. Within eight to sixteen hours after eating contaminated food, the following symptoms may occur: diarrhea, inflammation of the stomach and intestines, headache, cramps, and nausea without vomiting.

PREVENTION OF FOOD POISONING

Q. *How can food poisoning be prevented?*

A. Proper food handling and good hygiene can both limit bacterial contamination and slow the growth of any bacterial contamination already present. An individual should be aware of the following safety tips:

1. Buy canned foods without bulges. Bulging cans are a sign of food contamination.

2. Select frozen foods last at the supermarket and keep them frozen.

3. Read labels for dates that indicate freshness.

4. Purchase clean eggs that are free of cracks.

5. Refrigerate leftovers immediately after a meal.

6. Be sure the refrigerator is 40°F. or below and the freezer is 0°F. or below.

All leftover food should be placed in airtight containers and refrigerated.

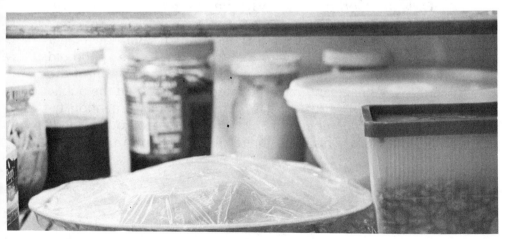

7. Refrigerate poultry and stuffing separately.

8. Use storage charts prepared by the U.S. Department of Agriculture for the recommended length of time to store food safely.

9. Clean the refrigerator, freezer, and other storage areas frequently.

10. Remember the two-hour rule: Two hours is the maximum total time any perishable food can be safely kept at room temperature. This includes shopping, preparation, and time on the table before consumption.

11. Thaw meat, fish, and poultry in the refrigerator. If necessary, hasten by placing under cool running water.

12. Wash knives, cutting board, and other utensils with soap and hot water after preparing raw meats to prevent cross-contamination of foods that may be eaten raw, such as salad greens and fruit.

13. Keep hot foods hot, above 140°F., and cold foods cold, below 40°F.

14. Follow safe recommendations of the U.S. Department of Agriculture for home canning.

15. Cook all home-canned foods for at least ten minutes to destroy any botulinum toxin.

16. Practice good personal hygiene.

SAFETY OF FOOD PRODUCTION SYSTEM

Q. *Is the food production system in the United states basically safe?*

A. Yes. Food in the United States is much safer now than it was in the past. People who want to return to the "good old days" do not understand what it was like at the turn of the century. Spoilage and microbe infestation exposed the public to the constant threat of gastroenteritis, not to mention typhoid, cholera, tuberculosis, and a variety of other food-borne diseases. This is no longer the situation in the United States.

The average per capita intake of food in this country is 1,400 pounds per year. Much of this food is purchased in the 250,000 retail food stores. More than 11,000 different food items can now be found in every supermarket at all times. Never in our history has the food supply been of such variety, quality, and quantity.

The food production system in the United States in the 1980s will be better than ever. It should not be feared but trusted.

Q. *If food in the United States is basically safe, why is there so much alarm from the popular press about the poisons in food?*

A. Some individuals have committed themselves to the cause of convincing American eaters that they are victims of overprocessed "junk foods" produced by uncaring food manufacturers. On the one hand, this cause is ego building because it creates much publicity. On the other hand, this cause is economic because such ideas sell well in the form of books and mailings.

The next time we wheel our grocery carts up and down the long aisles of the supermarket, we should stop for a moment and consider the variety and quality of food we have. Today, the food production system in the United States is the safest and best the world has ever known.

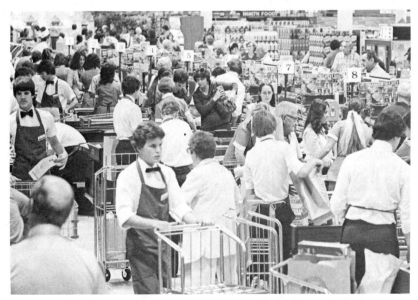

The tragedy is not that there are people who downgrade our food supply. There have always been fringe individuals, who, under the guise of consumer interests, make a career out of attacking the food supply. What is disappointing is the fact that the press and other news media give so much attention to unscientific statements. Steps in the right direction will not occur until concerned consumers inform their media representatives that they are interested in nutritional facts, not fiction.

COMMONSENSE NUTRITION

Q. *What is needed for the American people to have a rational view about food?*

A. According to Dr. Fredrick Stare, retired Professor of Nutrition at Harvard, the American public needs a refresher course in common sense. A lack of common sense is the primary reason that it is so much easier for pseudoscientists to sell food supplements than it is for ethical scientists with years of the best training available to convince people that optimum nutrition is obtainable from ordinary foods.

Every qualified nutritionist who speaks or writes about commonsense nutrition gets letters from belligerent people. These people insist that to be nutritious, apples must be grown without manufactured fertilizer, that vegetables must not be canned or frozen, that bread must not be white or enriched, that milk must not be pasteurized, that honey is more nutritious than white sugar, and many other variations of these themes.

"The food faddists and the health food stores," Dr. Stare points out, "promise what they call the *curative properties* of such things as honey and vinegar, organically grown vegetables, stone-ground flour, sunflower seeds, kelp, sea salt, and the trace minerals in the many odd combinations they so readily put together with added vitamins. We can't do it because we scientists use only information proved by scientific testing, . . . not the testimonials that are so often the support of the faddists."

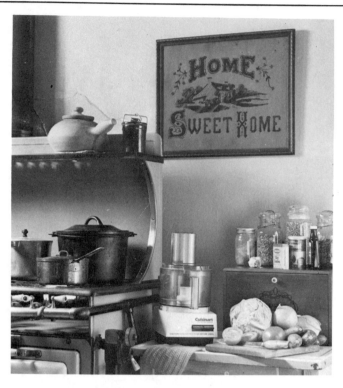

The wisdom passed down from Grandma's kitchen combined with today's science and technology yields commonsense nutrition.

In the United States today, it is not difficult to achieve optimum nutrition. Our supermarkets are stocked full of the most abundant, the most nutritious, the most economical, and the safest supply of food that any people has ever had. The quality of this food is produced by the same precise, scientific processes that have given us other advances. Would the average American let anyone send us back to the days of no automobiles, no washing machines, and no television? Of course not!

The time is ripe for Americans to return to commonsense nutrition. Let us accept, enjoy, and profit from the products of our food scientists. And let us banish food faddism, its magic, and its scare tactics to the distant past.

APPENDIXES

Appendix A: Recommended Dietary
Allowances—1980

Appendix B: Calorie Tables

Appendix C: Fourteen-Day, 1,000-Calorie Diet

Appendix D: Low-Calorie Recipes

Appendix A: Recommended Dietary Allowances—1980*

Age (years)	Weight (kg)	Weight (lbs)	Height (cm)	Height (in)	Protein (g)	Fat-Soluble Vitamins Vitamin A (RE)	Vitamin D (µg)	Vitamin E (mg)	Water-Soluble Vitamins Vitamin C (mg)	Thiamin (mg)	Riboflavin (mg)	Niacin (mg equiv)	Vitamin B6 (mg)	Folacin (µg)	Vitamin B12 (µg)	Minerals Calcium (mg)	Phosphorous (mg)	Magnesium (mg)	Iron (mg)	Zinc (mg)	Iodine (µg)
Infants																					
0.0-0.5	6	13	60	24	kg × 2.2	420	10	3	35	0.3	0.4	6	0.3	30	0.5	360	240	50	10	3	40
0.5-1.0	9	20	71	28	kg × 2.2	400	10	4	35	0.5	0.6	8	0.6	45	1.5	540	360	70	15	5	50
Children																					
1- 3	13	29	90	35	23	400	10	5	45	0.7	0.8	9	0.9	100	2.0	800	800	150	15	10	70
4- 6	20	44	112	44	30	500	10	6	45	0.9	1.0	11	1.3	200	2.5	800	800	200	10	10	90
7-10	28	62	132	52	34	700	10	7	45	1.2	1.4	16	1.6	300	3.0	800	800	250	10	10	120
Males																					
11-14	45	99	157	62	45	1000	10	8	50	1.4	1.6	18	1.8	400	3.0	1200	1200	350	18	15	150
15-18	66	145	176	69	58	1000	10	10	60	1.4	1.7	18	2.0	400	3.0	1200	1200	400	18	15	150
19-22	70	154	178	70	58	1000	7.5	10	60	1.5	1.7	19	2.2	400	3.0	800	800	350	10	15	150
23-50	70	154	178	70	58	1000	5	10	60	1.4	1.6	18	2.2	400	3.0	800	800	350	10	15	150
51+	70	154	178	70	58	1000	5	10	60	1.2	1.4	16	2.2	400	3.0	800	800	350	10	15	150
Females																					
11-14	46	101	157	62	46	800	10	8	50	1.1	1.3	15	1.8	400	3.0	1200	1200	300	18	15	150
15-18	55	120	163	64	46	800	10	8	60	1.1	1.3	14	2.0	400	3.0	1200	1200	300	18	15	150
19-22	55	120	163	64	44	800	7.5	8	60	1.1	1.3	14	2.0	400	3.0	800	800	300	18	15	150
23-50	55	120	163	64	44	800	5	8	60	1.0	1.2	13	2.0	400	3.0	800	800	300	18	15	150
51+	55	120	163	64	44	800	5	8	60	1.0	1.2	13	2.0	400	3.0	800	800	300	10	15	105
Pregnant					+30	+200	+5	+2	+20	+0.4	+0.3	+2	+0.6	+400	+1.0	+400	+400	+150	**	+ 5	+25
Lactating					+20	+400	+5	+3	+40	+0.5	+0.5	+5	+0.5	+100	+1.0	+400	+400	+150	**	+10	+50

The allowances are intended to provide for individual variation among most normal, healthy people in the United States under usual environmental stresses. They were designed for the maintenance of good nutrition. Diets should be based on a variety of common foods in order to provide other nutrients for which human requirements have been less well defined.

** Supplemental iron is recommended.

* From *Recommended Dietary Allowances*, 9th edition, 1980, National Academy of Sciences, Washington, D.C.

Appendix A: Recommended Dietary Allowances—1980 (continued)

Estimated Safe and Adequate Daily Dietary Intakes
of Additional Selected Vitamins and Minerals *

Vitamins

	Age (years)	Vitamin K (µg)	Biotin (µg)	Pantothenic Acid (mg)
Infants	0-0.5	12	35	2
	0.5-1	10-20	50	3
Children	1-3	15-30	65	3
	4-6	20-40	85	3-4
	7-10	30-80	120	4-5
Adolescents	11+	50-100	100-200	4-7
Adults	11+	70-140	100-200	4-7

Trace Elements

	Age (years)	Copper (mg)	Manganese (mg)	Fluoride (mg)	Chromium (mg)	Selenium (mg)	Molybdenum (mg)
Infants	0-0.5	0.5-0.7	0.5-0.7	0.1-0.5	0.01-0.04	0.01-0.04	0.03-0.06
	0.5-1	0.7-1.0	0.7-1.0	0.2-1.0	0.02-0.06	0.02-0.06	0.04-0.08
Children	1-3	1.0-1.5	1.0-1.5	0.5-1.5	0.02-0.08	0.02-0.08	0.05-0.1
	4-6	1.5-2.0	1.5-2.0	1.0-2.5	0.03-0.12	0.03-0.12	0.06-0.15
	7-10	2.0-2.5	2.0-3.0	1.5-2.5	0.05-0.2	0.05-0.2	0.1-0.3
Adolescents	11+	2.0-3.0	2.5-5.0	1.5-2.5	0.05-0.2	0.05-0.2	0.15-0.5
Adults	11+	2.0-3.0	2.5-5.0	1.5-4.0	0.05-0.2	0.05-0.2	0.15-0.5

Electrolytes

	Age (years)	Sodium (mg)	Potassium (mg)	Chloride (mg)
Infants	0-0.5	115-350	350-925	275-700
	0.5-1	250-750	425-1275	400-1200
Children	1-3	325-975	550-1650	500-1500
	4-6	450-1350	775-2325	700-2100
	7-10	600-1800	1000-3000	925-2775
Adolescents	11+	900-2700	1525-4575	1400-4200
Adults	11+	1100-3300	1875-5625	1700-5100

* Because there is less information on which to base allowances, these figures are not given in the main table of the RDA and are provided here in the form of ranges of recommended intakes. Since the toxic levels for many trace elements may be only several times usual intakes, the upper levels for the trace elements given in this table should not be habitually exceeded.

Appendix B: Calorie Tables*

MEAT GROUP

Calories

Beef

Beef and vegetable stew:

Canned	1 cup	185
Home made, with lean beef	1 cup	210
Beef potpie, baked	4½ inch, 8-ounce pie	560
Chili con carne, canned with beans	½ cup	170
Corned beef, canned	3 ounces	185
Corned beef hash	½ cup (about 3 ounces)	155
Dried beef, chipped	⅓ cup (about 2 ounces)	115

Hamburger broiled:

Regular ground beef	3 ounces	245
Lean ground round	3 ounces	185
Meat loaf	3 ounces	170

Oven roast, cooked, without bone:

(Cuts relatively fat, such as rib)

Lean and fat	3 ounces	375
Lean only	3 ounces	205

(Cuts relatively lean, such as round)

Lean and fat	3 ounces	165
Lean only	3 ounces	140

Pot roast, cooked, or braised beef, without bone:

Lean and fat	3 ounces	245
Lean only	3 ounces	165

Steak, broiled, without bone:

(Cuts relatively fat, such as sirloin)

Lean and fat	3 ounces	330
Lean only	3 ounces	175

(Cuts relatively lean, such as round)

Lean and fat	3 ounces	220
Lean only	3 ounces	160
Veal cutlet, broiled, without bone	3 ounces, trimmed	185

Lamb

Chop, broiled, without bone:

Lean and fat	3 ounces	305

* Courtesy of the United States Department of Agriculture.

Calories

Lean only	3 ounces	160
Roast, leg, cooked, without bone:		
Lean and fat	3 ounces	235
Lean only	3 ounces	160
Pork		
Bacon, broiled or fried	2 thin slices	60
	2 medium slices	90
Chop, cooked, without bone:		
Lean and fat	3 ounces	335
Lean only	3 ounces	230
Ham, cured, cooked, without bone:		
Lean and fat	3 ounces	245
Lean only	3 ounces	160
Roast, loin, cooked, without bone:		
Lean and fat	3 ounces	310
Lean only	3 ounces	215
Sausage		
Bologna	2 ounces	170
Liver sausage (liverwurst)	2 ounces	175
Pork sausage, bulk, cooked	2 ounces	270
Vienna sausage, canned	4 or 5	135
Variety and luncheon meats		
Beef heart, braised, trimmed	3 ounces	160
Beef liver, fried	3 ounces	195
Beef tongue, braised	3 ounces	210
Frankfurter, cooked	1	155
Boiled ham, luncheon style	2 ounces	135
Spiced ham, canned	2 ounces	165
Poultry		
Chicken:		
Broiled	¼ small broiler	185
Fried	½ breast	155
	1 whole leg	225
Canned, meat only	½ cup (about 3 ounces)	200
Poultry pie (with potatoes, peas, gravy)	4½-inch, 8-ounce pie	535
Turkey, roasted:		
Light meat	3 ounces	150
Dark meat	3 ounces	175

Calories

Fish and shellfish

Bluefish, baked	3 ounces..............	135
Clams:		
Canned	3 medium clams, and juice (3 ounces)......	45
Raw meat only	4 medium (3 ounces) ...	65
Crab meat, canned	½ cup (3 ounces)......	85
Fish sticks, breaded, deep fried	5 average	200
Haddock, fried in fat	3 ounces..............	140
Mackerel:		
Broiled	3 ounces..............	200
Canned	3 ounces..............	155
Oysters, raw	6 to 10 medium	80
Perch, fried in egg and breadcrumb coating	3 ounces..............	195
Salmon:		
Broiled or baked....................	3 ounces..............	155
Canned, pink.......................	³⁄₅ cup (3 ounces)......	120
Sardines, canned in oil.................	5 to 7 medium (3 ounces)	175
Shrimp, canned.......................	17 medium (3 ounces) ..	100
Tuna, canned in oil, drained.............	²⁄₅ cup (3 ounces)......	170
Eggs		
Fried in fat............................	1 large................	100
Hard or soft cooked, "boiled"	1 large................	80
Omelet, plain	1 large egg, milk, and fat for cooking..........	110
Poached.............................	1 large................	80
Scrambled in fat	1 large egg and milk....	110
Dry beans and peas		
Baked beans, in tomato sauce:		
With pork	½ cup	160
Without pork	½ cup	155
Limas, cooked.......................	½ cup, with liquid	130
Red kidney beans, canned or cooked	½ cup, with liquid	115
Nuts		
Almonds, whole	13 to 15	105
Brazil nuts	4	115
Cashews	5 large or 8 medium ...	60

Calories

Coconut:
Fresh, shredded	2 tablespoons	40
Dried, shredded	2 tablespoons	45
Peanuts.................................	2 tablespoons	105
Peanut butter	1 tablespoon	95
Pecans, halves........................	12 to 14	95

Walnuts:
Black, chopped......................	2 tablespoons	100
English halves	4 to 9	90

MILK GROUP

Milk:
Buttermilk.............................	1 cup.................	90
Condensed, sweetened, undiluted	½ cup	490
Evaporated, undiluted	½ cup	170
Half-and-half, milk and cream............	1 tablespoon	20
	1 cup.................	325
Skim, fresh or reconstituted dry	1 cup.................	90
Whole	1 cup.................	160

Cream:
Heavy whipping	1 tablespoon	55
Sour	1 tablespoon	30
	1 cup.................	505
Table, or coffee	1 tablespoon	30
Yogurt, made from	1 tablespoon	10
partially skim milk.....................	1 cup.................	120

Milk beverages:
Chocolate-flavored drink.................	1 cup.................	190
Chocolate milk	1 cup.................	210
Chocolate milkshake	12 ounces.............	520
Cocoa, all milk	1 cup.................	235
Malted milk	1 cup.................	280

Milk desserts:
Custard, baked	½ cup	140
Ice cream, plain	½ cup	145
Ice cream soda, chocolate	1 large...............	455

Calories

Ice milk:

Hard-serve	½ cup	110
Soft-serve	½ cup	130
Sherbet, fruit	½ cup	130

Cheese:

American, process	1 ounce	105
Blue	1 ounce	105
Cheddar, natural	1 ounce	115
	1-inch cube	70
	½ cup grated	225
Cottage, creamed	2 tablespoons	30
Cottage, not creamed	2 tablespoons	25
Cream	2 tablespoons	105
Parmesan, dry, grated	2 tablespoons	40
Swiss	1 ounce	105

VEGETABLE-FRUIT GROUP*

Vegetables (raw):

Cabbage (C):

Plain	½ cup, shredded	10
	3½ - x 4½-inch wedge	25
Coleslaw, with mayonnaise-type dressing	½ cup	60
Carrots (A)	5½ - x 1-inch carrot	20
	½ cup, grated	20
Celery	Two 8-inch stalks	10
Cucumber, pared	¾-inch slice	5
Lettuce	2 large leaves	10

Onions:

Young, green	6 small	20
Mature	2½-inch-diameter onion	40
	1 tablespoon, chopped	5
Peppers, green (CC)	1 medium	15
Radishes	4 small	5
Tomatoes (C)	1 medium	35

Vegetables (cooked, canned, or frozen):

Asparagus spears (C)	6 medium, or ½ cup cut.	20

* Good sources of vitamin C are marked (CC), fair sources are marked (C), and good sources of vitamin A are marked (A).

		Calories
Beans:		
Green lima	½ cup	90
Snap, green, wax or yellow	½ cup	15
Beets	½ cup, diced	30
Beet greens (A)	½ cup	15
Broccoli (A, CC)	½ cup flower stalks	20
Brussels sprouts (CC)	½ cup	20
Cabbage (C)	½ cup	20
Carrots (A)	½ cup diced	20
Cauliflower (C)	½ cup flower buds	10
Chard (A)	½ cup	15
Collards (A, C)	½ cup	30
Corn:		
On cob	One 5-inch ear	70
Kernels, drained	½ cup	70
Cress, garden (A, C)	½ cup	20
Kale (A, C)	½ cup	15
Kohlrabi (C)	½ cup	20
Mushrooms, canned	½ cup	20
Mustard greens (A, C)	½ cup	20
Okra	Four 3- x ⅝-inch pods	10
Onions, mature	½ cup	30
Parsnips	½ cup	50
Peas, green	½ cup	60
Peppers, green (CC)	1 medium	15
Potatoes:		
Baked (C)	2½-inch-diameter 5-ounce potato	90
Boiled	½ cup, diced	40
Chips	10 medium	115
French fries:		
Fresh cooked	Ten 2- x ½- x ½-inch pieces	155
Frozen	Ten 2- x ½- x ½-inch pieces	125
Hash-browned	½ cup	225
Mashed:		
Milk added	½ cup	60
Milk and fat added	½ cup	90
Pan-fried	½ cup	230
Sauerkraut, canned	½ cup	20

		Calories
Spinach (A, C)	½ cup	20
Squash:		
Summer	½ cup	15
Winter, baked, and mashed (A)	½ cup	65
Sweet potatoes (A):		
Baked in jacket (C)	5- x 2-inch, 6-ounce potato	155
Canned	½ cup	120
Honeydew melon (C)	2- x 7-inch wedge	50
Oranges (CC)	3-inch orange	75
Peaches	2-inch peach	35
Pears	3- x 2½-inch pear	100
Pineapple	½ cup, diced	40
Plums	2-inch plum	25
Raisins	½ cup	230
Tangerines (C)	2½-inch tangerine	40
Watermelon (C)	One 2-pound wedge	115
Fruit (cooked, canned, or frozen):		
Applesauce:		
Unsweetened	½ cup	50
Sweetened	½ cup	115
Apricots (A):		
Canned in water	½ cup, halves and liquid	45
Canned in heavy syrup	½ cup, halves and syrup	110
Dried, cooked, unsweetened	½ cup, fruit juice	120
Frozen, sweetened	½ cup	125
Berries:		
Blueberries:		
Canned in water	½ cup	50
Canned in heavy syrup	½ cup	130
Frozen, unsweetened	½ cup	45
Frozen, sweetened	½ cup	120
Raspberries, red frozen, sweetened	½ cup	120
Strawberries, frozen sweetened (CC)	½ cup	140
Cranberry sauce, canned	1 tablespoon	25
Figs, canned in heavy syrup	½ cup	110
Fruit cocktail, canned in heavy syrup	½ cup	100

Calories

Grapefruit, canned (CC):		
Water pack	½ cup	35
Syrup pack	½ cup	90
Peaches:		
Canned in water	½ cup	40
Canned in heavy syrup	½ cup	100
Dried, cooked, unsweetened	½ cup	110
Frozen, sweetened	½ cup	105
Pears, canned in heavy syrup	½ cup	100
Pineapple, canned:		
Crushed, in heavy syrup	½ cup	100
Sliced, in heavy syrup	2 small slices	90
Plums, canned in heavy syrup	½ cup	100
Prunes, dried, cooked: Unsweetened	½ cup	150
Sweetened	½ cup (8 or 9 prunes and 2 tablespoons liquid) . .	250
Rhubarb, cooked, sweetened	½ cup	190
Fruit juices:		
Cranberry juice cocktail	½ cup	80
Grape	½ cup	80
Grapefruit (CC):		
Fresh	½ cup	40
Canned:		
Unsweetened	½ cup	50
Sweetened	½ cup	65
Frozen concentrate, ready-to-serve:		
Unsweetened	½ cup	50
Sweetened	½ cup	55
Lemon	1 tablespoon	5
Lemonade, frozen concentrate, ready-to-serve	½ cup	55
Orange (CC):		
Fresh	½ cup	55
Canned, unsweetened	½ cup	60
Frozen concentrate, ready-to-serve	½ cup	55
Pineapple	½ cup	70
Prune	½ cup	100
Tangerine (C)	½ cup	50

BREAD AND CEREAL GROUP

Calories

Bread:

   1-pound loaf, 16 slices:

      Cracked wheat .... slice 75

      Raisin .... slice 75

      Rye................................... slice 70

      White................................. slice 75

      Whole wheat .... slice 70

   1-pound loaf, 20 slices:

      Cracked wheat .... slice 60

      Raisin .... slice 60

      Rye................................... slice 55

      White................................. slice 60

      Whole wheat .... slice 55

Biscuits, muffins, rolls:

  Baking powder biscuit .... 2½-inch-diameter biscuit 140

  Muffins:

      Bran .... 2¾-inch-diameter muffin 130

      Corn................................ 2¾-inch-diameter muffin 150

      English .... 3½-inch-diameter muffin 135

      Plain .... 2¾-inch-diameter muffin 140

  Rolls:

      Hamburger or roll frankfurter 1

                                  (18 ounces per dozen) .. 120

      Hard, round........................... 1 roll

                                  (22 ounces per dozen) .. 160

      Plain, pan .... 1 roll

                                  (16 ounces per dozen) .. 115

      Sweet, pan .... 1 roll

                                  (18 ounces per dozen) .. 135

Other flour-based foods:

  Cakes, cookies, pies..................... (See Desserts).

  Crackers:

      Graham .... 4 small, or 2 medium ... 55

      Matzoth .... 6-inch-diameter piece ... 80

      Oyster 10 45

      Pilot 1 75

      Rye wafers 2 45

Saltines	Two, 2 inches square ...	35
Soda	Two, 2½ inches square	50
Doughnuts:		
Cake-type, plain	1 average	125
Yeast-leavened, "raised."	2½- to 2¾-inch diameter	175
Pancakes (griddle cakes):		
Wheat	4-inch cake	60
Buckwheat	4-inch cake	55
Pizza, plain cheese	5½-inch sector of	
	14-inch pie	185
Pretzels	5 small sticks	20
Spoonbread	½ cup	235
Waffles	1 average	210
Breakfast cereals:		
Bran flakes	1 cup	105
Corn, puffed and presweetened	1 cup	115
Cornflakes	1 cup	95
Farina, cooked	1 cup	105
Oat cereal, puffed		
(mixture with mainly oat flour)	1 cup	100
Oatmeal or rolled oats, cooked	1 cup	130
Rice, puffed	1 cup	60
Rice, flakes	1 cup	115
Wheat, puffed	1 cup	55
Wheat, puffed and presweetened	1 cup	130
Wheat, shredded, plain	2 large, oblong biscuits	175
	1 cup spoon-size	160
Wheat flakes	1 cup	105
Grain products:		
Corn grits, cooked	¾ cup	95
Macaroni, cooked:		
Plain	¾ cup	115
With cheese	¾ cup	360
Noodles, cooked	¾ cup	150
Rice, cooked	¾ cup	140
Spaghetti, cooked:		
Plain	¾ cup	115
In tomato sauce, with cheese	¾ cup	195

		Calories
With meat balls	¾ cup	250
Wheat germ, toasted	1 tablespoon	25

BEVERAGES*

		Calories
Carbonated beverages:		
Cola-type	12-ounce can or bottle.	145
	8-ounce glass	95
Fruit flavors, 10-13	12-ounce can or bottle.	170
percent sugar	8-ounce glass	115
Ginger ale	12-ounce can or bottle.	115
	8-ounce glass	70
Root beer	12-ounce can or bottle.	150
	8-ounce glass	100

(Check the label of "low-calorie" drinks for the number of calories provided.)
Wines:

Table wines		
(Chablis, claret, Rhine wine, sauterne, etc.)	3-ounce glass	75
Dessert wines		
(muscatel, port, sherry, etc.)	3-ounce glass	125
Alcoholic beverages:		
Beer, 3.6 percent alcohol	12-ounce can or bottle.	150
Beer, 3.6 percent alcohol	8-ounce glass	100
Whiskey, gin, rum, vodka:		
70-proof	1½-ounce jigger	85
80-proof	1½-ounce jigger	95
86-proof	1½-ounce jigger	105
90-proof	1½-ounce jigger	110
100-proof	1½-ounce jigger	125

* [Not including milk and fruit juices.]

SOUPS*

		Calories
Bean with pork	1 cup	170
Beef noodle	1 cup	70

		Calories
Bouillon, broth, or consomme	1 cup	30
Chicken noodle	1 cup	60
Chicken with rice	1 cup	50
Clam chowder, Manhattan style	1 cup	80
Cream of asparagus	1 cup	85
Cream of mushroom	1 cup	135
Minestrone	1 cup	105
Oyster stew, homemade, with milk	1 cup, with 3 or 4 oysters	205
Split pea	1 cup	145
Tomato:		
Prepared with an equal volume of water	1 cup	90
Prepared with an equal volume of milk	1 cup	170
Vegetable with beef broth	1 cup	80

* Canned, condensed, prepared with equal volume of water unless otherwise stated.

FATS, OILS, AND RELATED PRODUCTS

		Calories
Butter or margarine	1 pat, 16 per ¼ pound stick	50
	1 tablespoon	100
Peanut butter	(See Meat Group; other high-protein foods.)	
Salad dressings:		
Blue cheese	1 tablespoon	75
French	1 tablespoon	65
Home-cooked, boiled	1 tablespoon	25
Low-calorie	1 tablespoon	15
Mayonnaise	1 tablespoon	100
Russian	1 tablespoon	75
Salad dressing, commercial-type		
plain	1 tablespoon	65
Thousand island	1 tablespoon	80
Salad Oil	1 tablespoon	125

DESSERTS AND OTHER SWEETS

Calories

Cakes:

Angel food	2-inch sector of 8½-inch tube cake	105
Boston cream pie	2-inch sector of 8-inch round layer cake	210
Chocolate cake, with chocolate icing	2-inch sector of 10-inch round layer cake	345
Fruitcake, dark	2-×2-×½-inch slice	140
Gingerbread	2-inch square	170

Plain cake:

without icing	3-×2-1½ inch slice.....	155
	2¾-inch-diameter cupcake	120
With chocolate icing	2-inch sector of 10-inch round layer cake	345
	2¾-inch-diameter cupcake	175
Pound cake	2¾-×3-×⅝-inch slice ..	140
Sponge cake	2-inch sector of 8½-inch tube cake	135
Yellow cake, without icing	2-inch sector of 8-inch round cake	205

Candies:

Caramels	3 medium	115
Chocolate creams.....................	2 or 3 small	110
Chocolate mints	2 small (1½-inches in diameter)...........	90
Fudge, milk chocolate, plain	1 ounce	120
Gumdrops	About 20 small (1 ounce)	100
Hard candy	1 ounce	110
Jellybeans............................	10	105
Marshmallows	4 large...............	90
Milk chocolate, sweetened	1-ounce bar	150
Milk chocolate, sweetened, with almonds ..	1-ounce bar	150
Peanut brittle........................	1 ounce	120

Calories

Other sweets:
  Chocolate:

Bittersweet	1-ounce square	135
Semisweet	1-ounce square	145
Chocolate syrup	1 tablespoon	50
Honey	1 tablespoon	65
Jam, jelly, marmalade, or preserves	1 tablespoon	55
Molasses	1 tablespoon	50
Syrup, table blends	1 tablespoon	55
Sugar, white or brown	1 teaspoon	15

Cookies:

Plain and assorted	3-inch cookie	120
Figbars	1 small	55

Pies:

Apple	⅛ of 9-inch pie	300
Blueberry	⅛ of 9-inch pie	285
Cherry	⅛ of 9-inch pie	310
Chocolate meringue	⅛ of 9-inch pie	290
Coconut custard	⅛ of 9-inch pie	270
Custard, plain	⅛ of 9-inch pie	250
Lemon meringue	⅛ of 9-inch pie	270
Mince	⅛ of 9-inch pie	320
Peach	⅛ of 9-inch pie	300
Pecan	⅛ of 9-inch pie	430
Pumpkin	⅛ of 9-inch pie	240
Raisin	⅛ of 9-inch pie	320
Rhubarb	⅛ of 9-inch pie	300
Strawberry	⅛ of 9-inch pie	185

Other desserts:

Apple betty	½ cup	170
Bread pudding, with raisins	½ cup	250
Cornstarch pudding	½ cup	140
Custard, baked	½ cup	140

Gelatin:

Plain	½ cup	70
With fruit	½ cup	80
Ice cream, plain	½ cup	145

Calories

Ice milk, hard-serve	½ cup	110
Prune whip	½ cup	100
Sherbet	½ cup	130
Tapioca cream pudding	½ cup	110

SNACKS AND OTHER "EXTRAS"

Bouillon cube	1 average	5
Corn chips	1 cup	230
Douhgnuts:		
Plain, cake-type	1 average	125
Yeast-leavened, "raised."	2½- to 2¾-inch diameter	175
French fries	Ten 2- x ½- x ½-inch pieces	155
Gravy	2 tablespoons	35
Hamburger (with roll)	2-ounce patty	265
Hot dog (with roll)	1 average	245
Olives:		
Green	4 medium, or 3 extra large	15
Ripe	3 small, or 2 large	15
Pickles, cucumber:		
Dill	1¾- x 4-inch pickle	15
Sweet	¾- x 1¾-inch pickle	30
Pizza, plain cheese	5½-inch sector of 14-inch pie	185
Popcorn, large kernel, popped with oil and salt	1 cup	40
Potato chips	10 medium	115
Pretzels	5 small sticks	20
Tomato catsup	1 tablespoon	15

Appendix C: Fourteen-Day, 1,000-Calorie Diet*

Some items are followed by numbers which correspond to numbered recipes found in Appendix D.

LOW CALORIE MENUS

Day 1

Breakfast. 210 calories:
1 orange or ½ cup orange juice; 1 egg (large) cooked to own preference (soft-boiled, poached, or fried in no-calorie vegetable cooking spray); 1 slice low-calorie bread or toast; 1 teaspoon low-calorie margarine or 1 tablespoon low-calorie jelly; no-calorie beverage (coffee, tea, water, soda).

Lunch. 400 calories:
Summer Salad[1]; 1 slice low-calorie bread; 4 oz. turkey; ½ cup skim or low-fat milk.

Dinner. 400 calories:
¼ cup cottage cheese; ½ cup asparagus; ¼ cup cooked carrots; 1 slice whole wheat bread; ½ cantaloupe or honeydew melon; 4 oz. leg of lamb, lean; no-calorie beverage.

Total Calories: 1,010

Day 2

Breakfast. 270 calories:
Grilled Swiss cheese sandwich: 1 oz. Swiss cheese; 1 tablespoon low-calorie margarine spread on 1 side of 2 slices low-calorie bread, grill using no-calorie vegetable spray; 1 cup tomato or V-8 juice; no-calorie beverage.

---

*From *How to Lose Body Fat,* by Ellington Darden, Winter Park, Florida: Anna Publishing, Inc., 1977, pp. 46–51, 58–61.

Lunch. 360 calories:
4 oz. lean ground hamburger; 1 slice low-calorie bread; 1 peach or plum; ½ cup boiled broccoli with 1 tablespoon lemon juice; no-calorie beverage.

Dinner. 370 calories:
½ cup skim or low fat milk; 1 slice low-calorie bread; 10 raw or steamed oysters (medium size), cocktail sauce, 2 tablespoons; baked apple; ½ cup cooked peas; no-calorie beverage.

Total Calories: 1,000

Day 3

Breakfast. 210 calories:
1 oz. cold cereal or ⅓ cup (uncooked) oatmeal; ½ cup skimmed milk or low fat milk; ½ grapefruit or ½ cup grapefruit juice; no-calorie beverage.

Lunch. 395 calories:
4 oz. roast beef on 2 slices low-calorie bread with 1 teaspoon mustard; ½ cup asparagus; ½ cup strawberries; 1 oz. farmer or pot cheese; no-calorie beverage.

Dinner. 375 calories:
4 oz. roasted turkey, meat only; ½ cup broccoli, with 1 tablespoon lemon juice; 1 slice rye bread; ½ cup cooked beets; ½ honeydew or cantaloupe melon; no-calorie beverage.

Total Calories: 980

Day 4

Breakfast. 205 calories:
½ cup fresh diced pineapple; 1 slice honey ham loaf; 1 slice low-calorie bread or toast; 1 teaspoon low-calorie margarine or 1 tablespoon low-calorie jelly; ¼ cup cottage cheese; no-calorie beverage.

Lunch. 385 calories:
3½ oz. tuna fish (oil-packed, drained); ½ cup cauliflower, boiled or raw; 1 slice low-calorie bread; 1 banana; ½ cup skimmed or low fat milk.

Dinner. 410 calories:
4 oz. roast beef, lean; 1 baked potato, without skin; 1 table-spoon sour cream; 1 slice low-calorie bread; ½ cup strawber-ries; no-calorie beverage.

Total Calories: 1,000

Day 5

Breakfast. 255 calories:
French Toast[2]; 1 teaspoon low-calorie margarine or 1 table-spoon low-calorie jelly; ½ cup apple juice; no-calorie bever-age.

Lunch. 315 calories:
Spinach Salad[3]; 2 tablespoons Italian low-calorie salad dress-ing; 1 slice pumpernickel bread; 1 teaspoon low-calorie mar-garine; 2 slices bacon cooked crisp; 5 prunes (dried); no-calorie beverage.

Dinner. 425 calories:
4 oz. veal loin chop for veal Parmesan[4]; ⅓ cup tomato sauce; ½ oz. Mozzarella cheese; ½ cup cooked cabbage; ¼ cup fresh sliced pineapple; ½ cup skimmed or low-fat milk.

Total Calories: 995

Day 6

Breakfast. 250 calories:
Dominique Egg[5]; 1 orange or ½ cup orange juice; 1 small sliced tomato; no-calorie beverage.

Lunch. 370 calories:
Honeydew-Turkey Salad[6]; ½ cup cauliflower with paprika; 1 slice whole-wheat bread; ½ cup skim or low-fat milk; no-calorie beverage.

Dinner. 380 calories:
½ cucumber, sliced; ¼ cup cottage cheese; 4 oz. flounder filet, with 1 tablespoon lemon juice; 1 slice rye bread; 1 ear of corn (medium size); 1 teaspoon low-calorie margarine; 1 apple; no-calorie beverage.

Total Calories: 1,000

Day 7

Breakfast. 235 calories:
1 cup tomato or V-8 juice; ½ cup flavored yogurt; 1 slice of low-calorie bread or toast; 1 teaspoon low-calorie margarine or 1 tablespoon low-calorie jelly; no-calorie beverage.

Lunch. 355 calories:
Beef Patty Parmesan[7]; Mushroom Parsley Salad[8]; no-calorie beverage.

Dinner. 405 calories:
½ cup skimmed or low-fat milk; 4 oz. roasted chicken, meat only; 1 cup spinach cooked with 2 tablespoons vinegar; 1 slice whole-wheat bread; ¼ cup unsweetened apple sauce; no-calorie beverage.

Total Calories: 995

Day 8

Breakfast. 265 calories:
1 oz. cold cereal or ⅓ cup (uncooked) oatmeal; ½ cup skimmed or low fat milk; 1 banana, no-calorie beverage.

Lunch. 370 calories:
Cucumber-Tuna Salad[9]; 2 carrots in sticks; 1 slice pumpernickel bread; 1 cup strawberries; $\frac{1}{2}$ cup skimmed or low fat milk; no-calorie beverage.

Dinner. 365 calories:
$\frac{1}{2}$ can beef consommé; 2 oz. broiled beef liver; $\frac{1}{2}$ cup cooked onions; 1 slice low-calorie bread; $\frac{1}{2}$ cup mashed acorn squash; $\frac{1}{2}$ cup grapes; no-calorie beverage.

Total Calories: 1,000

Day 9

Breakfast. 215 calories:
1 cup strawberries; 1 egg (large) cooked to own preference; 1 slice low-calorie bread or toast; 1 teaspoon low-calorie margarine or 1 tablespoon low-calorie jelly; no-calorie beverage.

Lunch. 370 calories:
$\frac{3}{4}$ cup cottage cheese; $\frac{1}{2}$ cup green beans (boiled or raw); 4 fish sticks; 1 sliced tomato; $\frac{1}{2}$ cup fresh pineapple slices; no-calorie beverage.

Dinner. 420 calories:
$\frac{1}{2}$ cup skimmed or low-fat milk; 4 oz. broiled lean beef steak; baked potato without skin; 1 tablespoon sour cream; $\frac{1}{4}$ cup blueberries.

Total Calories: 1,005

Day 10

Breakfast. 255 calories:
$\frac{1}{2}$ cantaloupe or honeydew melon; $\frac{1}{4}$ cup cottage cheese; 2 slices bacon cooked crisp; 1 slice low-calorie bread or toast; 1 teaspoon low-calorie margarine or 1 tablespoon low-calorie jelly; no-calorie beverage.

Lunch. 375 calories:
Pineapple Chicken Salad[10]; 2 lettuce leaves; 1 slice whole wheat bread; ½ cup skimmed or low-fat milk.

Dinner. 360 calories:
4 oz. steamed scallops; 1 slice pumpernickel bread; 1 tomato, broiled slices; ½ cup frozen French-cut green beans; 1 sectioned orange with ⅓ cup black raspberries; no-calorie beverage.

Total Calories: 990

Day 11

Breakfast. 210 calories:
1 apple; 1 oz. American processed cheese melted on 1 slice low-calorie bread (broiled); no-calorie beverage.

Lunch. 365 calories:
4 oz. canned salmon; 1 slice low-calorie toast; 1 pear; ½ cup winter squash, mashed; no-calorie beverage.

Dinner. 415 calories:
½ cup skimmed or low-fat milk; ½ cup green pepper, sliced; ½ cup beets; ¾ cup broiled mushrooms; 1 slice whole-wheat bread; 3 oz. fried beef liver, ½ cup cherries; no-calorie beverage.

Total Calories: 990

Day 12

Breakfast. 250 calories:
Scrambled Egg Special[11]; 1 slice low-calorie bread or toast; 1 teaspoon low-calorie margarine or 1 tablespoon low-calorie jelly; 4 oz. fresh diced pineapple; no-calorie beverage.

Lunch. 385 calories:
5 oz. lamb loin chop, broiled; ½ cup unsweetened apple-sauce; 1 cup cauliflower (boiled or raw) with ¼ cup American cheese, melted; 1 slice pumpernickel bread; ½ green pepper, 5 radishes; ½ cup skimmed or low-fat milk.

Dinner. 365 calories:
¼ cup cottage cheese; ¾ cup hot V-8 juice; 3½ oz. broiled trout; 1 slice low-calorie bread; ½ cup cooked cabbage; no-calorie beverage.

Total Calories: 1,000

Day 13

Breakfast. 280 calories:
Potato Pancakes[12]; 1 tablespoon sour cream; ½ cup tomato or V-8 juice; no-calorie beverage.

Lunch. 360 calories:
Oyster Spinach Soup[13]; 5 saltine crackers; 1 tomato, sliced; 2 oz. cottage cheese; no-calorie beverage.

Dinner. 360 calories:
½ cup skimmed or low-fat milk; Fried Chicken[14]; ½ cup asparagus; 1 tangerine, sectioned; no-calorie beverage.

Total Calories: 1,000

Day 14

Breakfast. 255 calories:
1 orange in sections with ½ cup blueberries; 1 oz. cold cereal or ⅓ cup (uncooked) oatmeal; ½ cup simmed or low-fat milk; no-calorie beverage.

Lunch. 255 calories:
Shrimp cocktail; 12 medium/large shrimp, 3 tablespoons cocktail sauce; Broccoli-Tomato Salad[15]; ½ cup green grapes; no-calorie beverage.

Dinner. 410 calories:
¼ cup cottage cheese with 1 peach sliced; 4 oz. broiled chopped lean sirloin; 1 slice whole-wheat bread; ½ tomato, sliced; no-calorie beverage.

Total Calories: 1,005

Appendix D: Low-Calorie Recipes

1. Summer Salad:

1 cup lettuce, shredded; 1 tomato, sliced; ¾ cup yellow crook-necked squash, sliced; ¼ cup green onion, sliced; dressing—1 tablespoon salad seasonings, Italian spice seasoning, and salt and pepper, plus 2 tablespoons vinegar. Mix all vegetables together. Top with dressing.

2. French Toast:

Dip two slices of low-calorie bread in mixture of 1 beaten egg, pinch of cinnamon, ⅛ teaspoon vanilla extract, and artificial sweetener. Using no-calorie cooking spray, brown bread on both sides. Top with low-calorie margarine, low-calorie jelly, or more cinnamon.

3. Spinach Salad:

1 cup torn spinach; ½ cup sliced mushrooms; ¼ cup sliced purple onions; 2 tablespoons toasted sesame seeds. Mix vegetables together. Sprinkle sesame seeds over top.

4. Veal Parmesan:

4 oz. lean veal; ½ oz. Mozzarella cheese, sliced; ⅓ cup tomato sauce. Heat tomato sauce in saucepan using preferred seasoning. Fry veal in no-calorie cooking spray. When done, turn heat off, add cheese to veal, and cover until melted. Pour tomato sauce over top and serve.

5. Dominique Egg:

Spread 1 slice low-calorie bread with 1 teaspoon low-calorie margarine. Cut a 2-inch hole in middle of bread. In skillet, using no-calorie vegetable spray, brown both slices of bread. Then crack egg into hole of bread and cook until ready. Top egg with circle of toast.

6. Honeydew-Turkey Salad:

$\frac{1}{2}$ honeydew melon, cubed; $\frac{1}{2}$ cup turkey, cubed; $\frac{1}{2}$ cup celery, sliced; 1 tablespoon onion, diced; 2 tablespoons low-calorie French dressing. Mix ingredients and top with French dressing.

7. Beef Patty Parmesan:

4 oz. lean hamburger; $\frac{1}{2}$ oz. Mozzarella cheese, sliced; $\frac{1}{3}$ cup tomato sauce. Heat tomato sauce in saucepan using preferred seasoning. Fry hamburger in no-calorie cooking spray. When done, turn heat off, add cheese to burger, and cover until melted. Pour tomato sauce over top and serve.

8. Mushroom-Parsley Salad:

$\frac{1}{2}$ cup mushrooms, sliced; $\frac{1}{8}$ cup parsley; $\frac{1}{8}$ cup radishes, finely sliced; $1\frac{1}{2}$ cups mixed greens (endive or bibb lettuce); pinch of basil, salt and pepper; 2 tablespoons low-calorie Italian dressing or wine vinegar. Combine ingredients, add seasonings, and top with dressing.

9. Cucumber-Tuna Salad:

1 small cucumber; $\frac{1}{3}$ can or 2 oz. tuna fish; $\frac{1}{4}$ cup shredded processed American cheese; $\frac{1}{8}$ cup chopped celery; 1 large hard-boiled egg, chopped; 1 tablespoon sweet pickle relish; 1 teaspoon onion, minced; $\frac{1}{2}$ teaspoon lemon juice; paprika; salt and pepper. Cut cucumber in half lengthwise and scrape out seeds. Cut a small slice from bottom of cucumber so it won't rock. Combine all ingredients and place in cucumber shells. Chill. Sprinkle with paprika and salt and pepper and serve. Makes 2 servings, 135 calories each.

10. Pineapple-Chicken Salad:

$\frac{1}{2}$ cup chicken, cubed; $\frac{1}{8}$ cup fresh pineapple, diced; $\frac{1}{2}$ red-skinned apple, diced; $\frac{1}{4}$ cup celery, diced; 2 tablespoons raisins; salt and pepper; 1 tablespoon sour cream. Combine all ingredients, toss, and chill. Serve on salad greens.

11. Scrambled Egg Special:

1 large egg, beaten; 1 tablespoon skimmed or low-fat milk; 1 tablespoon green onion, sliced; 1 slice honey ham loaf (cut into bite-size pieces). Stir all ingredients together and scramble using no-calorie cooking spray.

12. Potato Pancakes:

1 egg, beaten; 2 tablespoons skimmed or low-fat milk; 1 cup shredded potato; 2 tablespoons onion, diced; $1\frac{1}{2}$ tablespoons flour; $\frac{1}{4}$ teaspoon salt; $\frac{1}{8}$ teaspoon pepper. Combine egg and milk; add shredded potato and onion and mix. Then add flour, salt, and pepper and mix well. Using large skillet or electric griddle and no-calorie cooking spray, drop mixture by the spoonful (makes 3 to 4). Cook slowly until well browned and crisp. Turn and brown other side. Top with either sour cream or unsweetened applesauce.

13. Oyster-Spinach Soup:

1 cup skimmed or low-fat milk; 1 can condensed cream of chicken soup; 1, 10-oz. package frozen creamed spinach; 1, 8-oz. can of oysters, undrained; $\frac{1}{2}$ cup dry white wine; pepper; lemon slices. In a large saucepan stir milk into soup. Remove spinach from plastic pouch and add to soup. Cook and stir over medium heat, breaking up spinach until it is thawed. Simmer uncovered 10 minutes stirring occasionally. Stir in oysters, wine, and pepper. To serve, garnish with lemon slices. Makes 4 servings.

14. Fried Chicken Special:

½ chicken breast; salt and pepper; ⅛ cup bread crumbs. Season chicken breast with salt and pepper. Brown using no calorie cooking spray. Sprinkle half of bread crumbs on one side. Turn 5 minutes later and sprinkle the rest on. Cook until done.

15. Broccoli-Tomato Salad:

1 cup fresh broccoli flowerets; 2 tablespoons sour cream; dash of curry powder, dry mustard, seasoned salt, and pepper; 1 tomato, sliced. Cook broccoli in boiling salted water 3 to 4 minutes. Let cool. Combine sour cream and seasonings; pour over broccoli and stir to coat. Chill 2 to 3 hours. Add sliced tomato and serve on lettuce leaves.

bibliography

Alexander, Marie M., and Stare, Fredrick J. *Your Diet: Health Is in the Balance.* Washington: The Nutrition Foundation, Inc., 1979.

Appledorf, Howard. "Nutritional Analysis of Foods from Fast-Food Chains," *Food Technology* 28: 50–55, April 1974.

Arlin, Marian. *The Science of Nutrition.* New York: Macmillan Publishing Co., Inc., 1977.

Astrand, Per-Olaf, and Rodahl, Kaare. *Textbook of Work Physiology.* New York: McGraw-Hill, 1977.

Barrett, Stephen (editor). *The Health Robbers.* Philadelphia: George F. Stickley, Publishers, 1980.

Beller, Anne Scott. *Fat and Thin.* New York: Farrer, Straus and Giroux, 1977.

"Bread: You Can't Judge a Loaf by Its Color," *Consumer Reports* 41: 256–260, May 1976.

Briggs, George M., and Calloway, Doris H. *Bogert's Nutrition and Physical Fitness.* Philadelphia: W. B. Saunders Co., 1979.

Clydesdale, Fergus M., and Francis, Frederick J. *Food, Nutrition & You.* Englewood Cliffs, New Jersey: Prentice-Hall, Inc., 1977.

Cureton, Thomas K. *The Physiological Effect of Wheat Germ Oil on Humans in Exercise.* Springfield, Illinois: Charles C. Thomas, Publisher, 1972.

Darden, Ellington. *The Complete Encyclopedia of Weight Loss, Body Shaping, and Slenderizing.* King of Prussia, Pennsylvania: Westgate Press, Inc., 1980.

Darden, Ellington. *The Nautilus Book: An Illustrated Guide to Physical Fitness the Nautilus Way.* Chicago: Contemporary Books, Inc., 1980.

Darden, Ellington. *How to Lose Body Fat.* Winter Park, Florida: Anna Publishing, Inc., 1977.

Darden, Ellington. *Nutrition and Athletic Performance.* Pasadena, California: The Athletic Press, 1976.

Deutsch, Ronald M. *The Fat Counter Guide.* Palo Alto, California: Bull Publishing Co., 1978.

Deutsch, Ronald M. *The New Nuts Among the Berries.* Palo Alto, California: Bull Publishing Co., 1977.

Deutsch, Ronald M. *The Family Guide to Better Food and Better Health.* New York: Bantam Books, Inc., 1973.

Federal Trade Commission. *Advertising and Labeling of Protein Supplements.* Washington, D.C.: Government Printing Office, January 15, 1979.

Federal Trade Commission. *Protein Supplement Health Hazards and Marketing Deceptions: A Staff Report to the Federal Trade Commission.* Washington: Government Printing Office, August 8, 1975.

Hall, Richard L. "Safe at the Plate," *Nutrition Today* 12: 6–15, November/December 1977.

Hall, Richard L. "Food Additives," *Nutrition Today* 8: 20–28, July/August 1973.

Hamilton, Eva May, and Whitney, Eleanor. *Nutrition Concepts and Controversies.* St. Paul: West Publishing Co., 1979.

Institute of Food Technologists' Expert Panel on Food Safety and Nutrition. *Dietary Salt.* Chicago: Institute of Food Technologists, January 1980.

Institute of Food Technologists' Expert Panel on Food Safety and Nutrition. *Food Colors.* Chicago: Institute of Food Technologists, July 1980.

Institute of Food Technologists' Expert Panel on Food Safety and Nutrition. *Sugars and Nutritive Sweeteners in Processed Foods.* Chicago: Institute of Food Technologists, May 1979.

Institute of Food Technologists' Expert Panel on Food Safety and Nutrition. *The Risk/Benefit Concept as Applied to Food.* Chicago: Institute of Food Technologists, March 1978.

"Is Vitamin C Really Good for Colds?" *Consumer Reports* 41: 68–70, February 1976.

Jukes, Thomas H. "Carcinogens in Food and the Delaney Clause," *Journal of the American Medical Association* 241: 617–619, February 9, 1979.

Jukes, Thomas H. "The Predicament of Food and Nutrition," *Food Technology* 33: 42–51, October 1979.

Jukes, Thomas H. "How Safe Is Our Food Supply?" *Archives of Internal Medicine* 138: 772–774, 1977.

Kuntzleman, Charles T. "Dispelling Sauna Mythology: Not All Is as It Steams," *Science Digest* 87: 11–15, May 1980.

Kuntzleman, Charles T. *The Exerciser's Handbook.* New York: David McKay Co., Inc., 1978.

Lamb, Lawrence E. "Salt: Your Vital Sodium and Potassium Balance," *The Health Letter* 10, #12: 1–4, December 23, 1977.

Labuza, Theodore P. *The Nutritional Crisis: A Reader.* St. Paul: West Publishing Co., 1975.

Martin, Ethel A., and Coolidge, Ardath A. *Nutrition in Action.* New York: Holt, Rinehart, and Winston, 1978.

Mayer, Jean. *A Diet for Living.* New York: Pocket Books, 1977.

McNutt, Kristen W., and McNutt, David R. *Nutrition and Food Choices.* Chicago: Science Research Associates, Inc., 1978.

Melnick, Daniel. *A Teaching Manual on Food and Nutrition for Non-Science Majors.* Washington: The Nutrition Foundation, Inc., 1979.

National Research Council, Food and Nutrition Board: Recommended Dietary Allowances. Ninth revised edition. Washington: National Academy of Sciences, 1980.

Nelson, Ralph A. "What Should Athletes Eat? Unmixing Folly and Facts," The Physician and Sportsmedicine 3: 67–72, November 1975.

Nelson, Dale O. "Idiosyncrasies in Training and Diet," Scholastic Coach 30: 32–34, May 1961.

"Nutrition and Physical Fitness: A Statement by the American Dietetic Association," Journal of the American Dietetic Association 76: 437–443, May 1980.

Nutrition for Athletes: A Handbook for Coaches. Washington: American Alliance for Health, Physical Education, and Recreation, 1971.

"Nutrition Misinformation and Food Faddism, A Special Supplement," Nutrition Reviews 32: 1–73, July 1974.

Rayner, Clair. Everything Your Doctor Would Tell You If He Had the Time. New York: G. P. Putnam's Sons, 1980.

Robertson, Laurel; Flinders, Carol; and Godfrey, Bronwen. Laurel's Kitchen: A Handbook for Vegetarian Cookery and Nutrition. Petaluma, California, Nilgiri Press, 1976.

Ryan, Allan J. "Anabolic Steroids Are Fool's Gold." Paper presented at the 64th Annual Meeting of the Federation of American Societies for Experimental Biology, April 15, 1980.

Ryan, Allan J. "Severe Muscle Cramps After Prolonged Stressful Exercise," Journal of the American Medical Association 217: 1973, 1971.

Scrimshaw, Nevin S., and Young, Vernon R. "The Requirements of Human Nutrition," Scientific American 235: 50–64, September 1976.

Stare, Fredrick J., and Whelan, Elizabeth M. Eat OK—Feel OK! Food Facts and Your Health. North Quincy, Massachusetts: The Christopher Publishing House, 1978.

Steben, R. E.; Wells, J. C.; and Harless, I. L. Testing the Effects of Bee Pollen," Track Technique 64: 2046–2047, June 1976.

Stern, Judith S. and Denenberg, R. V. *How to Stay Slim and Healthy on the Fast-Food Diet.* Englewood Cliffs, New Jersey: Prentice-Hall, Inc., 1980.

Tannenbaum, Steven R. "Ins and Outs of Nitrites," *The Sciences* 20:15–20, January 1980.

"The Selling of H$_2$0," *Consumer Reports* 45: 531–538, September 1980.

Trager, James. *The Belly Book.* New York: Grossman Publishers, 1972.

"Unsugared Facts About Fructose, the Sweeter Sweetener," *Changing Times* 34: 48–50, June 1980.

"Vitamin E: What's Behind All Those Claims for It?" *Consumer Reports* 38: 60–66, January 1973.

"Yogurt: Will It Keep You Fit?" *Consumer Reports* 43: 7–12, January 1978.

index